Hidden Secrets of Super Perfect Health at Any Age

Hidden Secrets of Super Perfect Health at Any Age

Five Simple Proven Steps To Slow the Aging Process or Reverse it by Twenty Years

William L. Fischer

Fischer Publishing Corporation
Canfield, Ohio 44406

Hidden Secrets of Super Perfect Health at Any Age

Five Simple Proven Steps To Slow the Aging Process or Reverse it by Twenty Years

Copyright © 1985 by William L. Fischer

All Rights Reserved

No part of this book may be copied or reproduced in any form without the written consent of the publishers

ISBN: 0-915421-03-8

Library of Congress Catalog Number: 85-080558

Printed in the United States of America

Dedication

This book is affectionately dedicated to the millions of individuals and families who wish to take more responsibility for their own good health and well-being.

Mother always said: "Don't eat that junk; it isn't good for you." "Dress warmly; it's cold outside." "Clean up your plate; you need your greens." "It's a beautiful day! Go outside and play. You need some exercise."

Mother didn't know it, but she was practicing the very finest form of preventive medicine. The best preventive medicine in the world is merely using your own good common sense *to take care of yourself.*

It is my hope the contents of this book will provide you with a strong foundation for the time-honored practice of thoughtful preventive medicine. I believe good nutrition, natural foods and exercise suited to the age and condition of the individual are the bedrock on which to build your program of *Self-Care Health-Care*. I like to think mothers everywhere agree!

CONTENTS

Disclaimer

This book is informational only and should not be considered as a substitute for consultation with a duly-licensed medical doctor. Any attempt to diagnose and treat an illness should come under the direction of a physician. The author is not himself a medical doctor and does not purport to offer medical advice, make diagnoses, prescribe remedies for specific medical conditions or substitute for medical consultation.

Neither the author nor the publisher has any interests, financial or otherwise, with any of the manufacturers, distributors, retailers or other providers of any of the products referred to herein.

Foreword

The mythical "Fountain of Youth" has been sought by mankind since time began. Although we must accept the fact that this miraculous fountain does not exist, we can institute measures to slow down the aging processes.

Many of Grandmother's simple homemade recipes, rediscovered and revived, can better our health and improve the quality of our lives. Natural remedies show us the way to life extension and increased physical strength.

Hidden Secrets of Super Perfect Health at Any Age by William L. Fischer has come at exactly the right moment. In this modern world, more and more individuals are seeking ways to improve their life expectancy. The author, devoted to promoting the idea of natural health-care, tells us in plain, understandable language of amazing findings supporting the use of simple measures which can do just that. In my opinion, following the recommendations related in this book may result in significant longevity.

The benefits of these measures are within everyone's reach. They are not only instructively presented, but are documented by scientific evidence and testimonials of individuals who have successfully used them. *Hidden Secrets of Super Perfect Health* also presents the history of the methods presented and reports on recent scientific investigations. This book is a trustworthy guide to renewed health, vitality and well-being.

The first chapter reports on rebound exercise, called "rebounding" for short. In rebounding, all cells of our body are exercised at increased gravity force. What do we do when our hands are numb with cold in the winter? We swing them vigorously to enhance the bloodflow and increase the circulating action of the heart. Consider the lymphatic system which functions without the propelling action of a pump. Rebounding stimulates this vital bodily function. It's just like shaking fluid in a bottle to completely wet the inner surface. Rebounding is a fascinating and effective principle!

In the chapter on garlic, the author states his grandmother was right about the healing power of this odiferous herb. He must have read my thoughts! Anyone involved in holistic and preventive medicine will confirm the benefits of garlic. Not only has scientific research proven the efficacy of this plant, whose fame dates back to nearly 4000 years B.C., but individuals around the world who use garlic daily report incredible benefits.

In *Hidden Secrets of Super Perfect Health,* the author tells of one of the oldest of the natural nutritive products, bee pollen. Bee pollen is a complete food containing all elements man needs to survive and is a superior vitamin/mineral source from the beehive as well. Try bee pollen with your breakfast, instead of a laboratory manufactured pill. We can rely on the never-failing instincts controlling all nature. The bees know what's good and healthy and they're good natured enough to allow us to participate. Let's do it! The benefits are incalculable.

Dr. Rinse is a classic example of a man who followed St. Luke's injunction: "Physician, heal thyself." After a devastating heart attack, Dr. Rinse developed a completely natural formula that brought him back to perfect health. The Dr. Rinse Formula has since been used successfully around the world and offers an amazing healing potency. Many seriously ailing have regained their health and strength by taking Dr. Rinse's formula regularly.

Constipation is an all-too common malaise nowadays and is the cause of many secondary ailments. Instead of using—or often abusing—laxatives, *Hidden Secrets of Super Perfect Health* recommends a variety of natural remedies combined in a formula which can be prepared at home by anyone. All can benefit.

Man is justifiably proud of on-going achievements in the treatment of illness. But unfortunately, we sometimes tend to identify health-care with impressive chemical laboratories that turn out all manner of potions and pills which are willingly swallowed by the sick. We must remember, however, that it was Mother Nature herself who gave the clues. We steal her recipes, alter them slightly, make big profits and poison ourselves with the laboratory additives. Why don't we just go back to the original sources which offer an abundance of valuable, nonpoisonous products, ideal for holistic healthcare?

Hidden Secrets of Super Perfect Health recognizes the overwhelming trend back to natural self-care health-care growing by leaps and bounds around the world today and gives valuable recommendations anyone may use to relieve a number of common ailments and thereby improve the quality of their health. All recommendations are well-founded and clearly presented.

I wish this major contribution to holistic health care all the success it so richly deserves.

Dr. nat. sci. Hans L. Mennicken, N.D.

Preface

HIDDEN SECRETS OF SUPER-PERFECT HEALTH

By: William L. Fischer

Dear Friends:

Twelve years ago when I first began publishing and offering affordable little books with simple ways to better health each of us can practice in our daily lives, I could not know what blessings this activity would bring to me personally. Your letters have warmed and enriched my life—and I thank you.

So many wonderful people have taken the time to sit down and write me of their experiences after reading and following the suggestions in one book or another, I feel I now have many good friends scattered across the country. A number of you have been so impressed by a particular book, you have ordered extra copies for family and friends. And some of your letters expressed gratitude so beautifully I confess to becoming a little choked-up and misty-eyed.

As your publisher, I have a responsibility to you, my friends, that I take very seriously. Many writers come to me with manuscripts that are unsuitable or of no substance, manuscripts which would betray the trust you have in me. You have my promise I will never publish such books.

I have been reading your letters for a long time now and what I hear more and more is that you want to know how to take a more active part in keeping or regaining robust good health, that feeling of being on top-of-the-world, eager and raring to go every morning!

Self-Care Health-Care seems to be what you're looking for and it is to this very worthwhile goal that my newest series of books is dedicated.

In this opening book of the series, I tell you about some ancient ideas for keeping fit that work. I introduce you to "The World's Only Perfect Food," relished by the original Greek Olympians, some current Gold Medal winners, and President Ronald Reagan.

I bring to your attention an "old wive's tale" that has now been confirmed as very effective preventive-medicine by modern science. Together, we explore a new type of exercise so gentle and simple even a great-grandmother can benefit—and yet so challenging a young marathon runner might select this as a method of training for a hard race.

In addition, this book provides you with a secret formula developed by a doctor for cleaning out clogged arteries. In fact, this incredible formula can actually prevent hardening of the arteries, a major cause of heart disease. And, I have included a kitchen-recipe you can put together yourself with simple ingredients that will cure the most stubborn case of constipation ever recorded *and* prevent this potentially dangerous and certainly agonizing problem from ever troubling you again!

This book includes some inspiring stories of others who have regained their health by using the methods laid out for you in the following pages—in some cases, in spite of having been given a discouraging prognosis by the orthodox medical establishment.

If you and your family and friends are well and happy, I'm so glad! Perhaps some of these simple ideas will protect your health. If you are suffering ill health—or a member of your family is suffering with ill health—I wish you the same happy results others have had.

William L. Fischer
Canfield, Ohio 44406

SECTION I

An Introduction to the Miracles of

REBOUNDING

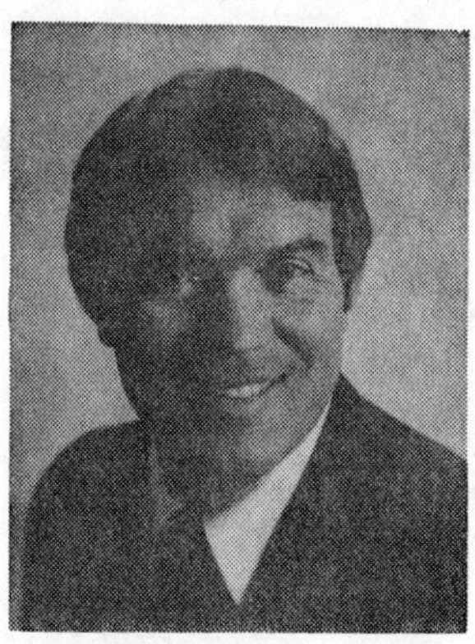

Al Carter has qualified twice for Olympic Competition. He has won 44 Gold Medals and 6 Silver Medals in amateur competition as All-Around Gymnastic Champion of five different states. He has won three state wrestling championships. Al Carter doesn't jog and he has never lifted weights—yet he can do over 100 one-arm pushups without stopping!

Al Carter is the designer of The Rebound mini-trampoline unit, founder of Rebound Dynamics, and developer of the Rebound Exercise program which has brought new life and hope to countless devotees of rebounding world-wide. Rebounding is unique among exercises in that it can be both gentle and simple enough for a wheelchair patient and yet so challenging and strenuous an Olympic athlete might select it as a training aid. But the real beauty of rebounding is that individuals of any age and in any state of health can benefit!

REBOUNDING FOR BOUNDLESS BENEFITS

LAVERNE GROFF: HER STORY—"And they were married and lived happily ever after." Some fairy tales end that way, but the first seven years of my married life were a nightmare. I was in and out of hospitals more times than I like to remember. Less than a year after we were married, my husband rushed me to the hospital. My ovary had ruptured, I was bleeding internally, and the doctor said I was lucky to be alive. He had to remove half the ovary. Less than a year later, the same thing happened and I was back in the hospital for the removal of the other half of the same ovary.

A short nine months later, my other ovary ruptured and I was back in the hospital for my third operation. Each time I was admitted, bigger tumors and cysts began appearing.

In the recovery room, after my third operation, my heart stopped. The quick action of the doctors and nurses started it beating again. A week later, after various tests, the doctor told me they had found something else that had to be corrected.

After all these operations and so much convalescence time, I was unable to exercise. A short time after my last operation, my body just gave up. My nerves and muscles no longer functioned. I practically became a vegetable and couldn't talk for over two months. Someone had to feed me. I didn't have the strength to lift my arms and walking was impossible. My back was so weak I was always in pain. I began seeing a chiropractor and he really helped me. But as I began to learn to walk all over again, I was in constant pain from my back and my operations.

I prayed desperately, "Oh, Lord. Isn't there any hope for me?"

Shortly thereafter, my husband and I were introduced to rebound exercise while attending one of Dr. Corwin West's self-help clinics. Dr. West told me he had seen only one other person in worse physical condition in his many years of practice. But we took home a rebounder and determined to follow Dr. West's instructions.

At first I had to sit on the rebounder with my feet on the mat while my husband bounced. We did this for a few minutes several times each day. In a few weeks, I tried it by myself, sitting at first, then finally standing alone. As the months went by, I could feel my strength coming back. It was almost like climbing out of a dark grave into a meadow full of flowers. I was alive! My pain was disappearing. Not only were my arms and legs getting stronger, I could actually feel my insides getting stronger! Neither my family doctor nor my chiropractor could believe I was the same person!

After using the rebounder for a year, we wouldn't give it up for all the world. We also have the most wonderful news that could have ever happened to us. We are expecting our first baby! The doctor said if I hadn't developed so much strength in my insides, I could never be carrying this baby. Considering the fact that we did it with only half an ovary, we thank our dear Lord each day for leading us to rebounding and Dr. West.

I want everyone to know this rebounder is the best thing I have ever found for eliminating pain without pills. I am now up to 15 minutes of running and jumping on the rebounder several times a day and I feel just wonderful!

NOTE: LaVerne Groff gave birth to a six-pound baby a few months after writing her story for us. Because of her previous health problems, her doctors were on the lookout for complications. Instead, after keeping the baby in the hospital for five weeks as a precaution, they found the baby perfectly healthy and normal. Both mother and baby are happy and healthy and *home*!. Needless to say, dad is just as proud as a peacock!

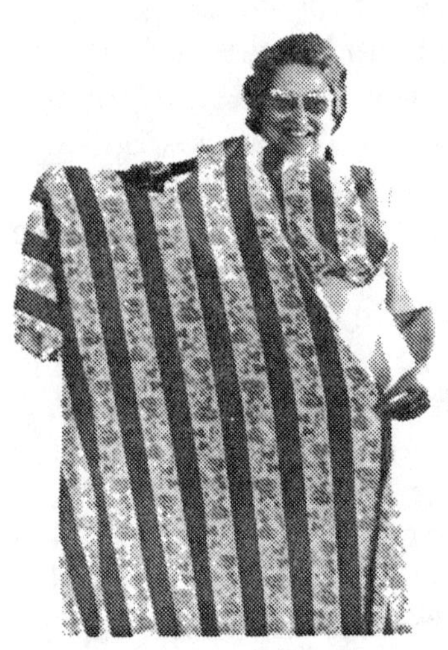

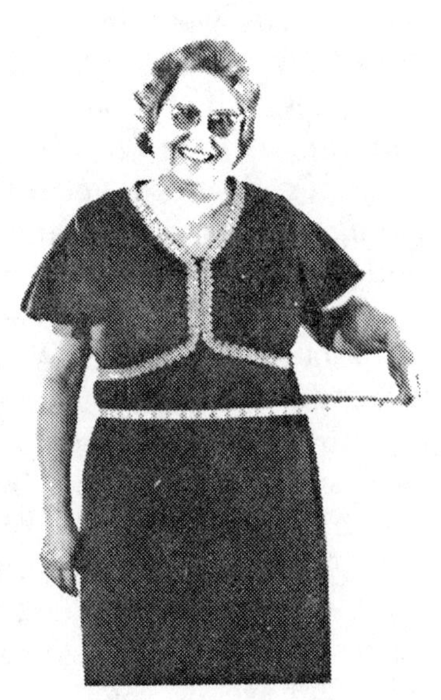

Dorothy Ross: "After just 2 1/2 months, my backaches were gone. I had no more headaches, arthritis or bursitis pain and I went from a size 24 1/2 to an 18 1/2!"

WALT & DOROTHY ROSS: THEIR STORY–My name is Dorothy Ross and I'm not going to tell you how old I am, but I'm the proud grandmother of 21 beautiful grandbabies . . . and I feel as good right now as I did when I was 35, but that wasn't true last February or the hard years before.

Early in the 1960s, I was hospitalized for a pinched nerve. The x-rays showed early arthritis had settled in my spine. My arthritis spread to my right knee and both ankles. I had bursitis in the right shoulder and both hips.I suffered with a constant backache and always felt completely exhausted. Other problems plagued me, too, and the years seemed long with headaches, high-blood pressure, ringing in my ears and poor balance and I literally cried many nights with pain from my bursitis. Walt finally bought me a four-inch foam pad to cover the mattress, but the pain was still excruciating.

Mind you, all of this had been going on for years on end and I was constantly under a doctor's care. He told me I was "just getting old and had to expect this sort of thing," but I didn't want to agree with him.

Walt had severe and painful problems, too. He suffered a heart attack, was found to be a diabetic a few years ago and had *four* cancer surgeries last year—two of them within 28 days! I worried about Walt and he worried about me. We were both discouraged and sick and tired of being sick and tired. We began to pray together for some form of exercise or *something* that would help us overcome our physical problems so we could enjoy life again.

After a week of fervent prayer, Walt brought home a rebounder. He was excited, but I was skeptical. For three days I watched him bounce for thirty seconds at a time. Each day he seemed brighter and had more energy. His disposition turned happy and sunny and he literally began to whistle while he worked, something I hadn't heard for a long, long time. I was just about ready to decide "it was all in his mind." I couldn't believe a simple exercise like bouncing could make such a change in any length of time, let alone just three days.

With his example, I tried to use the rebounder, but couldn't keep my balance. Walt held my hands to steady me and for three days, morning and evening, I did 25 counts of a gentle bounce. Sure enough—I began to feel better, too! In two weeks, my blood pressure dropped 30 points, I had more stamina, I lost 8 pounds and began to sing while I worked—literally sing! Life took on a whole new outlook. I had hurt for so long and been tired for so long, I had actually forgotten how it felt to feel really good—no, really *great*!

After just 2 1/2 months, my backaches were gone. I had no more headaches, arthritis or bursitis pain. The leg and foot cramps that woke me up every night disappeared. I lost 20 pounds (!) and went from a size 24 1/2 to an 18 1/2. I heal more quickly and sleep soundly for the first time in years! No wonder I feel as good as I did when I was 35!

And listen to what rebounding has done for Walt! His stamina and recuperative powers have reached phenomenal dimensions. He lost 18 pounds and within a short period of time, could run a mile. His cholesterol level, which had always been too high and was the cause of his heart attack, is 10 points below normal. His heart-rate dropped 8 beats per minute and is now slow and steady. His eyesight has cleared. He now drives and watches television without glasses. The doctor says Walt is now in better physical condition than any time since he has known him and he might even be completely free of diabetes within a few months!

Are we thrilled and excited and happy to share the unbelievable benefits of the rebounder? You bet! Our whole life has changed for the better. We are happier, healthier, busier and eager for each new day.

Both of Walt's doctors were so impressed with his rapid recovery and incredible physical progress with the rebounder, it took only 15 seconds for each of them to decide they needed one themselves!

IN THE WORDS OF HARRIS NELSON: Harris Nelson of Hollywood, California—70 years young—sums up the benefits of rebounding in inimitable style.

"All you have to do is bounce on the rebounder, very easily at first (convalescents can sit on it), and it's astounding how it massages every organ in the body. The results have been fantastic! The concept is new. Bouncing puts all the cells in the body under stress. In defense, they fortify themselves, strengthening their walls. They become stronger and *so do you*!. It's as simple as that! And it works!

"I need only six hours of sleep at night now—and no tossing as before—I wake up refreshed. No more getting up nights. Stress and anxiety reduced 100%. Cough gone. Arthritis gone. I can eat anything now, even before going to bed and I don't wake up dizzy and nauseated at four in the morning because of my heart problem. NO ANGINA PAINS! I never enjoyed better regularity or elimination—it's perfect. I have renewed zip and vitality. I've lost eight pounds and no dieting. All muscles are firmer. My "pot belly" is reduced 1 1/2 inches. I can read music faster. My mind reacts quicker—and I'm sure it corrected disorders I wasn't even aware of. Plus, plus, plus!

"All this—and why? Better circulation. Stronger lung power and a stimulated lymphatic system (your toxic poison and waste removal system)—action and movement. Exercise! And, happy day, I can do it all while watching television. No special garb, no sweat!

"And it's done all this for me in less than four months, exercising just five minutes twice a day. That's all you need to keep fit!"

AN EXPLANATION OF REBOUNDING

Just what is a rebounder anyway? Basically, the rebounder is a mini-trampoline sized for personal indoor use. A circular unit of varying size, it stands 12″ off the floor and the plasticized mat is suspended on a series of sturdy springs around its circumference.

In 1979, Albert E. Carter of *Gymnastics Fantastics,* the trampolining family which tours the country putting on incredible exhibitions of trampolining, published a book called "The Miracles of Rebound Exercise." Al himself attended Oklahoma State University on full scholarship for his wrestling prowess and has qualified twice for Olympic Competition. He was also All-Around Gymnastic Champion of five different states and boasts 44 Gold Medals and 6 Silver Medals in amateur competition before turning professional 18 years ago. Pretty impressive credentials.

Al Carter, as a professional trampolinist, has been personally involved with rebound exercise for over 30 years. He is an author, a lecturer and is considered a physical fitness expert. Al is the world's foremost authority on trampolining—rebound exercise—called the "most efficient, effective form of exercise yet devised by man."

When Al was first introduced by a friend to the household rebounder, he admits to being skeptical. (After all, Al Carter is used to highly professional and costly trampolining equipment, much too large for a living room.) Al remembers wondering how in the world anyone could jump on a trampoline in the average house without either denting the ceiling with his skull or hitting the floor through the mat, probably both. But he was impressed with the quality of the mini-trampoline and his words explain it best:

"It stood less than a foot off the ground on six round

chrome legs and looked as if it were trying to hide by blending in with all the other furniture. I went over and picked it up, turned it over and attacked its soft underbelly fully expecting to find a fatal flaw. Surprisingly, I was impressed with the solid, quality construction. I carefully studied the stitching; it was strong. And I had to admit the springs were uniquely triangulated and of better quality than those on my professional trampoline. Each spring protected the other by not allowing its neighboring spring to extend to maximum length. I turned the unit over, set it on its sturdy chrome legs, stood back and looked at its profile."

Ah-ha, I thought, "There's the flaw. It's too low. No adult could bounce on that without hitting the floor. In fact, the fabric would probably rip out with any amount of use at all. I took off my shoes and stepped in the middle. It was surprisingly resilient. After a couple of quick, easy bounces, I put my heels together and thrust into the mat. My attack was met by an equal and opposing force that catapulted me into the air—and I didn't hit the floor.

"I felt a curious rising anticipation. It was as if someone had read my mind and developed this machine according to my specifications. This was possibly the first individualized rebound machine to meet my rigid requirements."

In a word, Al was "sold" on the unit and has become its strongest advocate.

Mind you, I have always believed the best way to find out about something is to go straight to the source. Albert E. Carter is unquestionably THE source for information on rebounding and its boundless benefits. We are indebted to Al for all the material on rebounding in these chapters, most of which has come straight from his book. After we prepared this necessarily brief "condensation," it was submitted to Al for editing and updating. Because we know many of you will recognize rebounding just might be the answer to your prayers, as it has been for so many others, we list Al Carter's address at the close of this section so you can go straight to the source for the name of a Rebounder distributor in your area—and to purchase Al's book, "The Miracles of Rebound Exercise," the in-depth explanation of rebounding, known as the "bible" to enthusiastic rebounders everywhere.

THE HOW & WHY OF REBOUNDING

The common denominator of all forms of exercise is opposition to the gravitational pull of the earth. Think about it. Every exercise ever devised depends on gravity to make it effective. Push-ups, chin-ups, sit-ups, leg-lifts, weight-lifting—all depend on opposing the force of gravity with a specific part of the body. The aerobic exercises, such as walking, jogging or running, and the currently popular "jazzercise" classes, depend on the gravitational pull of the earth to be effective. Even in swimming, it is gravity that makes the water dense enough to create resistance to the musculature of the swimmer.

Gravity is the most important and constant physical force of our existence. You have to have opposition to develop strength. Where there is no opposition, there is no strength. To use the law of gravity for strength, we must oppose it.

Gravity, of course, is so much a part of our lives we don't think much about it. In addition, two other forces govern the way we get around—acceleration and deceleration. Gravity is a constant factor, but we can control acceleration and deceleration and harness them for our betterment. With the rebounder, we line up acceleration and deceleration with gravity. This is the purpose of the rebounder.

As we stand still on a rebounder, every cell in the body is opposing gravity. Your bathroom scale can be used as a "G" (gravity) meter. Place your bathroom scale on the rebounder and stand upon it. The scale registers one G force as long as you stand still. However, something fascinating happens when you start to move up and down. At the bottom of the bounce, you no longer weigh one G—you weigh *more* because the scale registers the combined forces of gravity *plus* deceleration when your body stops its downward thrust and acceleration when the expanded springs of the rebounder contract and force your body back up.

Acceleration + Deceleration + Gravity = Greater G Force! Even without allowing your feet to leave the rebounder mat, your G force increases to approximately 125%. It is vitally important to realize that every cell in your body is directly affected by that 25% increase in G force. Each cell is individually stressed by an increase of 25%.

If you ask a doctor, physical therapist or coach for the formula to strengthen your cells, the answer would be, *"Controlled stress, below the rupture threshold, times repetition."* Bouncing on a rebounder stresses every cell over and over again approximately 100 times per minute. Remember, every cell in your body has the unique ability to automatically adjust to its environment. By stressing every cell over and over again, every cell will begin to adjust to a greater G force and thereby become stronger. If the word "stress" bothers you, think "exercise" instead. But this is one instance where "stress" is good for your body.

Other forms of exercise only oppose gravity, and thereby strengthen, *part* of your body. But if you oppose gravity with the added force of acceleration and deceleration created by rebounding, *you strengthen every cell in your body all at once.* This, in a nutshell and oversimplified, is the amazing theory of rebound exercise. You can now begin to understand *why* rebounding has to be the most efficient, effective form of exercise yet devised by man.

There is three times more lymph fluid in the body than there is blood. What is "lymph?" Lymph is the clear fluid that oozes over a cut once it stops bleeding. Lymph is water, nutrients on the way to the cells and waste byproducts excreted from the cells for disposal. Lymph fluid is in constant motion around all cells. Our cells are able to function better with fresh lymph filled with a proper concentration of oxygen, glucose, certain electrolytes, amino acids, protein, essential fatty acids, carbohydrates and hormones. When these vital substances replace the waste products of the cells—the toxins, poisons and trash that build up around inactive cells—we are healthier.

Because the lymph does not circulate with a pump system, as blood does, what moves it around? Lymph travels through our Auxiliary Circulating System, tubes whose cell walls are only one-cell thick. They reach nearly every part of the body. Where these tubes don't reach, there are minute passages where lymph can flow. The tiny lymph tubes are filled with millions of one-way valves. Lymph moves along on a pressure hydraulic system. Pressure built up below the valve causes it to open. Pressure above the valve keeps it closed. An increase in pressure causes the lymph to flow upward.

The lymphatic system has the responsibility of pulling out waste, toxins, poisons and extra-cellular trash from the body. Lymph fluid, filled with toxins, waste, excess protein and dead cellular particles, is sucked into the lymph tubes to be filtered by the spleen and the lymph nodes. The lymphatic system is our "vacuum cleaner," the garbage collector of the body.

Rebound exercise has been found the single most effective method of stimulating lymphatic circulation. Rebounding yields the greatest change in pressure for the least muscle effort. Why is that important? If our lymphatic system functions properly, we are healthy. If the lymph circulates improperly, we fall ill.

Every cell in the body is an "intelligent" entity in itself. Each cell has within its walls the complete blueprint of the entire body. Although every cell in the body owns its own copy of the blueprint, it only "reads" that part of the blueprint that has to do with its own function. A skin cell will always be a skin cell, a bone cell will always be a bone cell and a liver cell will always be a liver cell.

Red blood cells, the most abundant of all the body's cells, are adept at transporting oxygen from the lungs to the tissues. Their function makes it necessary that they be able to move around the cardiovascular system without attachments. Red blood cells make up about 25% of all the body's cells.

Because every cell in the body has the ability to automatically adjust to its own environment, any change in the environment stimulates that cell or group of cells. Each cell is made strong by the amount and type of stimulation it receives. The stimulation put on a cell comes from three sources: (1) atmospheric or environmental pressure; (2) the gravitational pull of the earth and (3) muscular activity. The greater stimulation applied to the cell, the stronger it becomes as it adjusts to its environment.

Rebound exercise is a method of stimulating every cell of the body simultaneously by increasing the G force applied to every cell. As we add the forces of acceleration and deceleration to gravity, every cell in the body begins to adjust automatically to its new environment.

MUSCLE STRENGTH & PHYSICAL FITNESS ARE NOT THE SAME—A study of the fitness, health and longevity of individuals over 100 years of age around the world, most of slight build best described as "wiry," revealed a very important common denominator. In every case, just getting through a normal day's work required great physical exertion. Using modern techniques, heart and lung function of these persons were monitored. Astoundingly enough, many of these people had "silent" cardiovascular diseases without exhibiting any of the usual symptoms such as shortness of breath, and high blood pressure—but had not succumbed to a heart attack! The inescapable conclusion was that the seeming harshness of their daily lives stressed each cell constantly, resulting in an individual able to withstand a normally lethal heart attack!

Muscles are communities of cells with one main responsibility—to contract upon demand, thereby moving a bone or organ. Muscles get their strength from the combined total strength of their individual cells. In order to strengthen a muscle, the cells of that muscle must be strengthened individually.

Body-builders, for instance, concentrate on strengthening and building their muscles. *A muscle may be strong, but the individual may not be fit or healthy.* If the necessary oxygen and nutrients are not available when the cell needs them, or if there are too many toxins, wastes and poisons around the cell, it is impossible for the cell to function properly and the muscle will quickly become fatigued.

Many people mistake the terms "strength" and "physical fitness." Physical fitness is a measure of circulation efficiency. Increase the circulation efficiency of the body's fluids—the lymph and the blood—and the body is then physically fit and the muscles are able to continue to work longer without fatigue.

Rebounding not only increases the strength of each muscle by increasing the G force repeatedly, but also increases the fitness of the body by improving the lymphatic and blood circulation servicing the muscle. Unless your aim is bulging biceps, physical fitness is more important to most of us than mere muscle strength.

How in the world do you exercise an internal organ?—By rebounding to exercise the *cells* that make up the organ, of course. In the same way we strengthen muscle, we can build stronger, more efficient vital organs.

Various organs within the body are responsible for controlling the homeostatic condition of the environment for the individual cell. Many hundreds of control mechanisms are necessary to control arterial pressure, oxygen concentration, carbon dioxide concentration and the rates of individual chemical reactions in the individual cells. Each cell of each organ has to "do its own thing" without interfering with the function of cells within other organs. And each organ must work in harmony with the others.

All control systems of the body have certain characteristics in common. Most body organs function by reacting to opposition of their neutral position. For example, if the extra-cellular fluid becomes unbalanced, the system controlling a group of organs initiates the changes that cause an opposite reaction. This keeps the environment of the cells that comprise the organs near a certain concentration, maintaining the necessary balance.

The stimulation of the rapid vertical movement of the body on a rebounder causes all vital organs to work harder at controlling the body's environment. Because the rebounder has cured many physical problems, many people call it a "miracle machine." But the rebounder is not the miracle—the body is. The rebounder merely assists the body's organs to function more efficiently.

REBOUNDING IS AEROBICS, PLUS—*Aerobics* is the term used to define the function of cells that need oxygen to burn nutrients to create energy. All cells need oxygen and are therefore aerobic. Any activity, including sleeping, needs oxygen.

The body is unable to store oxygen, but we are able to replenish our supply simply by breathing. The problem is not *supplying* the body with oxygen—it is *delivering* oxygen to the cells where it is needed.

Exercise that elevates the heart-rate stimulates the pumping action of oxygen-carrying blood to all parts of the body. Aerobic exercise delivers greater amounts of oxygen to all cells more efficiently. In addition, increased demands on the body's arteries improves their elasticity. To transport blood effectively, our arteries must contract their inside diameters. But our arteries have a tendency to harden and become less elastic as we age, making the necessary contractions difficult. Aerobic exercise

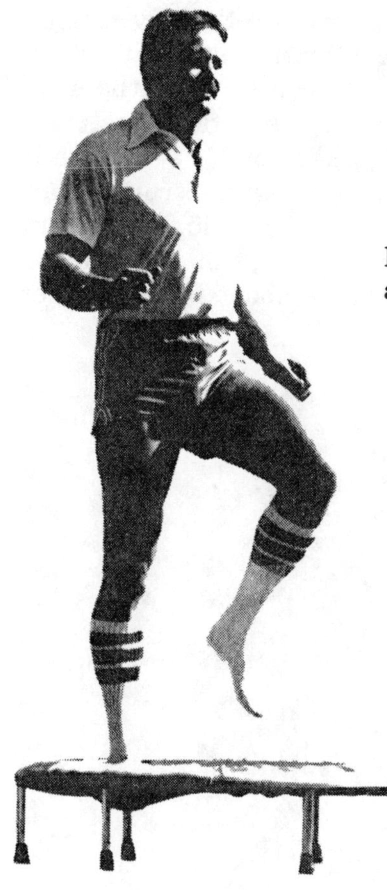

Randy Earl demonstrating the aerobic use of The Rebound.

reverses this trend, causing arteries to become more elastic and easier to contract.

Who needs aerobic exercise? We all do—but not the level of exertion which often accompanies the better-known aerobics such as walking, jogging, swimming, cycling and running. Many authorities caution that our bodies are not capable of coping with the shock and trauma caused by many of these activities.

However, the heart-rate drops after performing a good aerobic exercise for a few weeks. The heart muscle itself also increases in strength under controlled environmental stress, improving cardiac output. In other words, the heart can do more work with each beat, or the same work with fewer beats. The average American has a resting pulse rate in the neighborhood of 75. As a case in point for aerobics, both trampolinists and runners are famous for having pulse rates as low as 45. (Al Carter's resting pulse rate has been recorded as 39.) An individual with an efficient heart saves about fifteen million heart-beats per year!

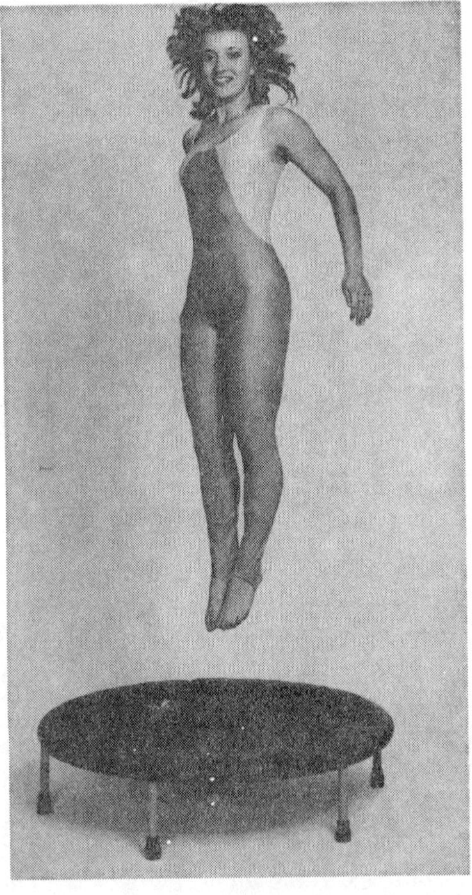

Wendie Carter.
(Al's daughter)
Girls just wanna
have fun!

The premise behind aerobics is to create increased oxygen circulation to the cells. But the *real* answer is *aerobics plus increased fluid circulation.* Any activity which increases oxygen circulation will also cause increased fluid circulation. In the study of aerobics, the benefits appear to be caused by more efficient oxygen consumption, when, in fact, the benefits of aerobic activity are actually a result of a *combination* of better lymphatic circulation, better delivery of nutrients by the blood, more efficient oxygen utilization from the lungs and even better elimination and digestion because of more efficient body fluid circulation.

Studies conducted at the University of California show maximum cardiovascular efficiency can be achieved by rebounding aerobically for two four-minute periods daily. Although it brings other benefits as well, rebounding for any longer than that will not improve heart efficiency noticeably. But the beauty of rebounding over running, the most popular aerobic exercise, is that rebounding doesn't foster "jogger's kidney," muscle strains, pulled ligaments or joint inflammation.

SURPRISE YOUR EYES—Who ever heard of exercising your eyes? In fact, most people are astounded to learn vision can be improved with exercise. We assume a person is born with "good" or "bad" eyes and nothing can be done about it. The idea of improving eyesight through exercise can be traced to the Egyptians, but we have become so convinced that we have no control over the condition of our eyes that we calmly accept the inconvenience.

You may be surprised to learn that the shape of the eyeball changes under stress, pressure, exercise, nutritional deficiencies, illness, shock or trauma. While examining over 30,000 eye patients per year, Dr. William W. Bates of the College of Physicians & Surgeons noticed some of his patients could see better on some occasions than others. He noted that far-sightedness and nearsightedness came and went on some of his patients, *contrary to everything he had been taught.* This led him to the logical conclusion that the eyeball must be able to change shape and could be influenced by emotional stress, strain and exercise.

How do we exercise the eye? Visual therapists have developed a number of eye exercises proven beneficial under specific circumstances and certainly any qualified ophthalmologist will be able to provide you with instruction. But where does rebounding fit into visual therapy?

The rebounder contributes more to the organization of visual perception than any other known device. Our control of movement comes from the visual mechanism, because the eyes are the primary "steering" machinery for all movements. Improved vision comes about when the millions of cells in the eyes and the muscles controlling the eyes are individually stimulated to do a better job because of increased stress.

Try rebounding and "see" for yourself.

I WANNA BOUNCE!

You have read the two preceding chapters with growing enthusiasm and now you're convinced that rebounding is the perfect exercise for you . . . and you're right. Rebounding is so incredibly versatile it *is* the perfect exercise for everyone and everyone can benefit. It doesn't matter whether you're a great grandparent, an infant or an athlete—or somewhere in between. Rebounding can be both gentle enough for a patient in a wheelchair and challenging enough for an athlete in training.

Rebounding is healthy exercise for the entire body, but a few cautions are in order. Injured cells, new cellular formations, aging cells and cells weakened by disease or disuse have a very low threshold. Some elderly or extremely inactive people may experience pain or swelling in their weaker parts after rebounding.

This does not mean that rebound exercise is not good for them. It merely means they should rebound with a gentler bounce, how gentle being determined by how weak their cells are. By *gradually* rebounding longer and harder, they will become stronger and increase their threshold to the point where they no longer have to worry about hurting something with the slightest amount of exercise.

Our bodies respond positively to challenge. The difference between our bodies and a mechanical device is that an automobile, for instance, deteriorates from wear and tear—but the body *improves* with use as long as the activity is not too violent.

When beginning any exercise program, be conservative. Do not over exert yourself. Build your endurance slowly. Rebound exercise is so easy that many beginners rebound too long the first time and feel it the next day. A consultation with your doctor is in order if you have any serious condition of ill health. However, rebounding is all it's said to be and the number of testimonials from enthusiastic rebounders is growing by leaps and bounds with glowing reports of ill health conquered.

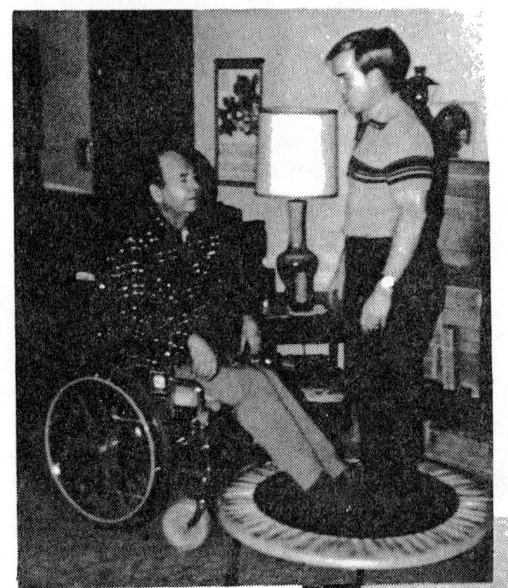

Al Carter (with Norman Nielson) demonstrating the early use of The Rebound with a wheelchair patient.

Al Carter (with Norman Nielson) demonstrating a more advanced program of rebounding for an incapacitated patient.

THE FACTS OF LIFE

Presented by Al Carter,
President of Rebound Dynamics, Inc.

FACT I. Most rebound units are not built well enough to support a consistent exercise program longer than 30 days.

FACT II. NASA has confirmed to Al Carter personally that Rebound Exercise is as much as *68% more efficient* than jogging.

FACT III. Rebound Exercise is fun, easy, convenient, economical and safe for most people.

FACT IV. Al Carter's company, *Rebound Dynamics,* has exclusive distribution rights to all copyrights owned by The National Institute of Reboundology & Health, which has published over 95% of all Rebound Exercise literature available.

FACT V. Rebound Exercise helps improve body balance, coordination, rhythm, timing and dexterity while building muscle strength.

FACT VI. Rebound Exercise is here to stay because it is *the most efficient and effective form of exercise* yet devised by man.

THE DECLINE & FALL OF THE DRUGSTORE REBOUNDER

In 1979, Al Carter's first book, *Miracles of Rebound Exercise,* introduced rebounding to a wildly enthusiastic general public and sales skyrocketed. All those with the nose for a fast-buck jumped on the bandwagon and cheap, shoddy rebounders flooded the marketplace.

By 1980, there were over 100 manufacturers trying to cash-in on the rebound exercise industry. If the nylon mat *looked* like expensive permatron, customers couldn't tell the difference—until a half hour after they started bouncing. Some never did figure out why rebounding didn't seem to do much for them. The trouble is that nylon, like plastic and canvas, stretches. Most of these good people who thought they caught a bargain had simply never experienced rebounding on the right kind of equipment. They didn't know the difference between the sluggish thud of feet on their unit and the exhilarating free springing mat of a good unit.

Thin metal frames, cheap springs that stretched-out or snapped and rubber leg tips that wore through in less than a month, damaging floors or carpet, made it easy to reduce the price still more. Most people couldn't tell the difference in the store anyway.

Then the mass merchandisers entered the market in a big way, awarding a manufacturing contract to the lowest-bidder, of course. The mass merchandisers weren't knowledgeable enough on the health benefits of rebounding to understand the necessity of a quality unit. They just wanted a piece of the mini-trampoline market pie like everybody else. The main function of the mass merchandisers is to sell product to the masses—and, at $49.00 per unit, they succeeded.

The next entries came from foreign shores. Made with cheap materials and even cheaper labor, the foreign manufacturers stole the market with units retailing in drugstores and even some supermarkets at $19.95 and most of the U.S. manufacturers went out of business. The price war on rebounders that Al Carter predicted two years ago had finally run its course.

More than a million and a half rebounders were sold in 1983. These figures were up by more than 33% over 1982 when an astounding 72 million dollars were spent by consumers on rebounders! In 1984, department stores, discount stores, sporting goods stores and drugstores accounted for more than 78% of all sales of rebound units. These are the rebounders disgusted consumers pitched into the trash when the springs were sprung or the legs broke off or the mat split. The original and dedicated U.S. manufacturers responsible for starting the industry took in only 13% of the sales volume. *Why?* Their actual construction costs were more than the cheap units' full retail price!

If you're one of the millions who got stuck with a piece of junk in the past and gave up on rebounding—or if you're new to this form of exercise—the best news of all is that Al Carter has personally supervised the design and construction of a rebounder which will meet or exceed the requirements of Certified Reboundologists all over the world! Called *The Rebound,* this unit retails for around $140 and is being manufactured in Taiwan in order to keep the price affordable.

Al tells me he has emphatically impressed on the factory that *quality* is essential. If manufactured in the U.S., the price would necessarily be around $250 retail for the same quality, but Al feels strongly it's vitally important to keep the cost of *The Rebound* within reach of all those who need it.

Al Carter has personally developed eleven specific exercises for the rebounder, one or more of them just right for you.. Space considerations prevent our showing the pictures and instructions you will find in his book, but the titles of each will give you an idea of the wide range possible on *The Rebound.*

They are: (1) Health Exercise, (2) Aerobic Exercise, (3) Strength Exercise, (4) Twist, (5) Dance, (6) Slalom, (7) Goose Step, (8) Sitting, (9) Sitting with Assistance, (10) Wheel Chair Rebounding, and (11) The "V" Bounce.

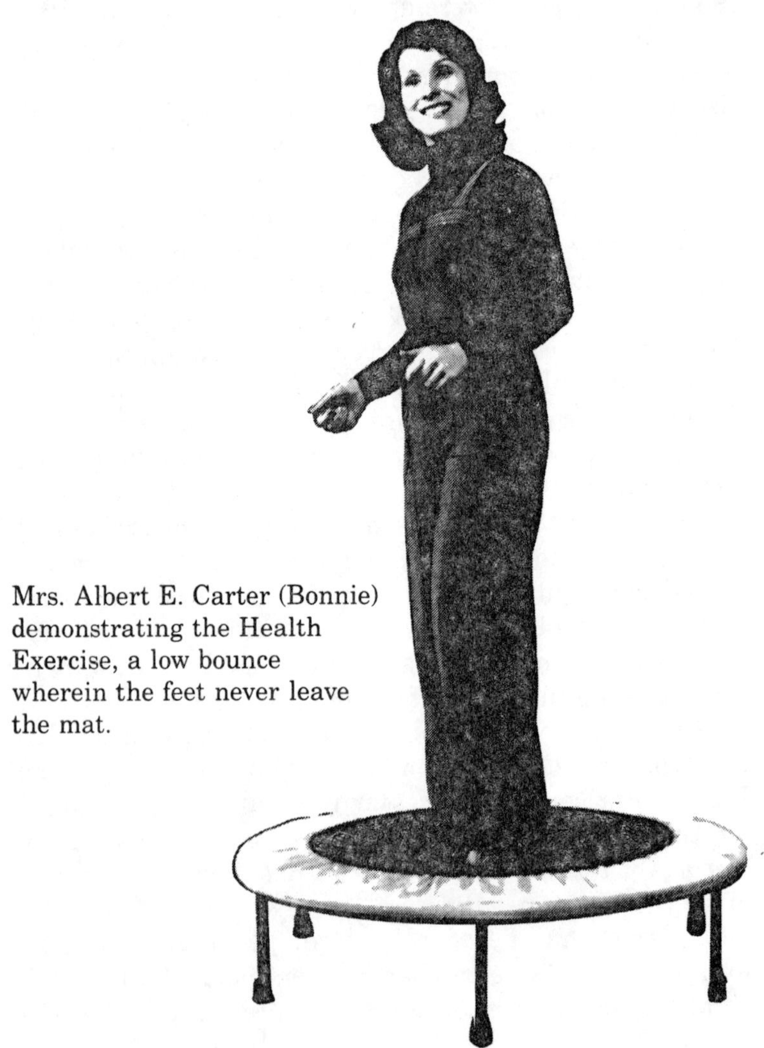

Mrs. Albert E. Carter (Bonnie) demonstrating the Health Exercise, a low bounce wherein the feet never leave the mat.

You will also find eye exercises, plus a method of improving memory and an explanation of how trampolining is a positive aid to education in schools.

You have nothing to lose but your aches and pains and excess weight. I strongly urge you to contact Al Carter for the name of your local Rebound distributor and to secure a copy of his book, *The Miracles of Rebound Exercise.* Incidentally, Al has another even more comprehensive book on rebounding in the works, so ask about it when you write or call. To contact Al, write or phone:

Mr. Albert E. Carter
REBOUND DYNAMICS, INC.
P.O. Box 5968F
Lynnwood, Washington 98036
(206) 771-1462

Great-Grandmother was Right about

GARLIC

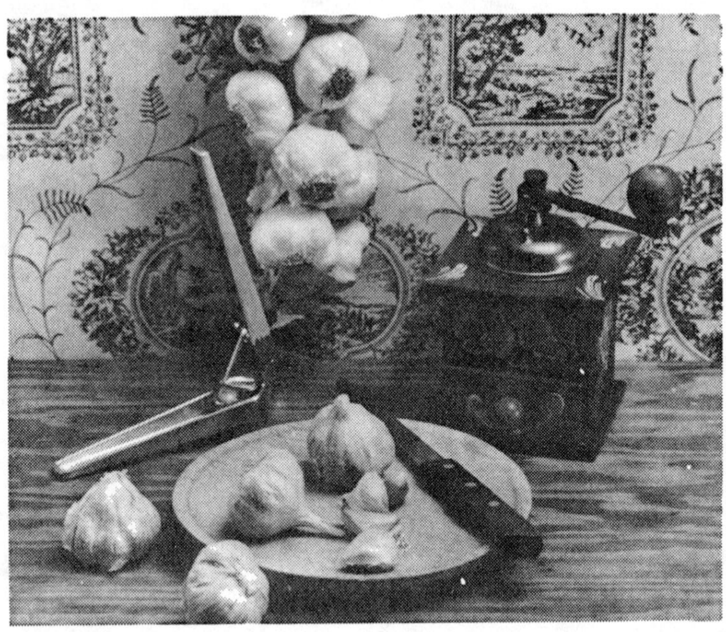

Modern science confirms that garlic is antiseptic, antibacterial, antifungal and bacteriostatic. Garlic, used by healers in over 5,000 years of recorded history, is effective against bronchial congestion, circulatory problems, heart disease and more—and may yet prove to be the cancer-preventive researchers all over the world have been searching for!

FOLK REMEDY REDISCOVERED

Science Finds Garlic a Possible Cancer Preventive—and More!

Deep in Germany's fabled Black Forest you come with surprise on a huge creaking old farmhouse that looks like it's been there forever, run down now, but still as friendly and welcoming as it was when I was a boy. The farm acreage has turned into a meadow overrun with parsley gone wild, as tall as my knee, the crisp curly green fronds swaying in the breeze very much like a green wheat field run riot.

On vacation last year, I trekked the old paths back to Grandfather and Grandmother's farm and was transported back in memory to green springs and golden summers when my grand and very important doctor father stayed behind in Heidelberg while mother and I summered at the farm.

As my eye wandered from the verdant green of the parsley, I saw the faint outline of Grandmother's kitchen garden and I was suddenly reminded of Brigetta, the hired girl. Brigetta was as hearty and healthy and happy and strong as the milk-cows she tended. She sang at the top of her voice and never minded having me skipping along at her heels. She told me with superstitious awe the legends of the Bavarian country folk—and she smelled as ripe as an old shoe from the cut clove of garlic she wore suspended on a string around her neck and the pungent breath she exhaled with gusto. The garlic, she promised me, would keep off the evil eye.

Grandmother, too, was a believer in the power of garlic. Not to ward off the evil eye, but as a medicament and health-protecting food. Every spring, without fail, the first sweet new butter coming from her cows eating the new shoots of grass was turned into her version of a "spring tonic."

As Brigetta churned the butter into nuggets, Grandmother took down a couple of bulbs of dried garlic from the braided string hanging near the kitchen fireplace and pounded them into a mash with her largest pestle in a big worn wooden bowl. When Grandmother had a smooth paste and the fumes were stinging all eyes, Brigetta scooped up a slab of the pale sweet butter and added it to the pounded garlic as Grandmother mixed it in.

When she was satisfied the garlic had permeated every smidgen of the butter, Grandmother then smoothed the aromatic mixture into a heavy crock and lowered it inside a larger crock with many pebbles in the bottom. Brigetta brought in icy-cold water from the well and poured it into the space around the smaller crock and popped on the heavy lid. The crock was kept in the cold-room in the earthen cellar and this primitive ice-chest kept the pungent mixture fresh all summer long.

Although my mother protested, Grandmother insisted, and even mother took a small tangy spoonful after noon supper every day, as we all did. I grew to relish the taste, but Mother rinsed her mouth with salt water and delicately chewed parsley to cleanse and sweeten her breath after downing her portion with an expression of distaste.

Grandmother maintained her pungent garlic paste was an aid to digestion and a sure way to stop a body from succumbing to the coughs, sore throats, colds and sniffles that were a part of life in our frigid winters. Although my scientific-minded father scoffed at such an old remedy, even he became convinced of the great benefits of this herb and became a strong advocate in later years. Thanks to Grandmother's garlic paste, I can testify I was always singularly free of any type of illness or respiratory distress throughout my childhood and sported outside all winter long in the chill air while many of my schoolboy friends sniffled and snuffled and were kept in by their anxious mothers.

Smiling at the thought of the little boy I had been and remembering that Grandfather died at 101 and Grandmother at an incredible 105, I determined to do a little research when I got home to find out if garlic does possess any of the powers Grandmother and Brigetta attributed to that singularly aromatic herb. Like so many other so-called "old wive's tales," I found there is a strong scientific basis for Grandmother's belief. It is very likely my grandparents owed the robust good health they enjoyed well past the Biblical "three-score years and ten" to their daily ration of garlic paste. Garlic *can* protect our health and assists in the cure of many and varied complaints as well.

GARLIC THROUGH THE AGES & AROUND THE WORLD

In 3748 B.C., Egyptian slaves working on the great pyramid of the Pharoah Cheops staged what was certainly the first sit-down strike in recorded history. Why? The slave-masters stopped their daily ration of garlic! This ancient herb was so highly regarded for its strengthening properties that the slaves risked death rather than be without it.

Ancient Vikings and Phoenicians never set their sails without a healthy supply of garlic on board—and probably avoided coming down with scurvy because of it. Early Chinese, Greeks and Romans used garlic to expel intestinal worms, a common and dangerous complaint of the times, relieve indigestion, heal skin rashes, treat respiratory problems and to stop infection in its tracks. In addition, garlic is thought by many to slow the aging process. In Bulgaria, even today, garlic is still chewed religiously by the general population—and many Bulgarians live active lives past 100-years of age.

Marco Polo, certainly one of the best-known explorers of medieval times and a very prolific and expressive writer, recorded his experiences in 13th century Cathay (China) for posterity. In his journal, Marco Polo noted that the higher castes of China ate meat preserved in several expensive special spices—but the poor had to be content with meat steeped in garlic juice! Knowing what we know today, we must conclude the poorer classes had the better of it.

In very early recorded history, the most notable uses of spices and herbs were in medicines, in holy oils, in unguents and as aphrodisiacs. Priests of many sects employed spices and herbs in incantations, rites and ritual worship. Difficult as it may be to believe, garlic was included in this distinguished company. Both the common bulb vegetables, garlic and onions, are pictured on many Egyptian monuments surviving the Pharoahs and are mentioned in many medieval sacred writings as well.

Lloyd J. Harris, in researching garlic, found the decadent Roman aristocracy used garlic because of its power to remove sexual inhibitions and maximize pleasure in sexual activity. Ancient rabbis decreed garlic should be eaten on the night of the Sabbath, the time devoted to marital enjoyment. Certain sex-abstaining religions prohibited the eating of garlic altogether because of the physical desire it creates.

A favored aphrodisiac found in centuries-old Hindu writings, currently enjoying a revival today, is the unlikely combination of garlic and roses! Proponents say this "magic potion" will increase sexual desire and performance, fade wrinkles to make you look years younger and melt away ugly fat bulges. To make the Garlic/Rose Elixir, peel one entire head of garlic and place all cloves (slightly crushed) in a large jar. Add raw natural honey (not the filtered supermarket variety), to cover. Next, take two handfuls of fresh-picked rose petals and crush them. Place the crushed rose petals in a teapot and fill with boiling water. Allow the petals to steep for ten minutes. Add the hot rose petal tea to the garlic-honey mixture slowly and stir gently to melt the honey. Permit the mixture to remain undisturbed for 48 hours for full potency.

Directions for use of this triple-threat "magic potion" are: To banish wrinkles, dilute three tablespoons of the Elixir with a little water and smooth on your face. Leave on for 20 minutes and rinse off with warm water. As a weight-loss appetite depressant, take one tablespoon (undiluted) immediately before eating. To heighten sexual pleasure, both partners should take one tablespoon of the potion (undiluted) immediately before indulging in sexual activity. Experts theorize that it is the phosphorus content of garlic which affects sexual excitability, causing instantaneous and prolonged arousal.

As a medicament, in 1897, master-herbalist W.T. Fernie wrote these words about garlic in his "Herbal Simples," an authoritative healing source of the day, "The bulb, consisting of several cloves, is stimulating, anti-spasmodic, an expectorant and diuretic. Garlic proves useful in treating asthma, whooping cough and other spasmodic afflictions of the chest. The pain of rheumatic parts may be much relieved by simply rubbing them with cut garlic."

Additional medicinal uses for garlic down through the ages have included tightening loose teeth, removing tartar deposits and the treatment of polio, tuberculosis, ear infections, open wounds, typhus, cholera—and even the Black Plague!

One tale told concerning garlic's amazing powers is purported to have happened during the Great Plague of France. Occurring in 1721, this plague was even more devastating than the better-known Plague of London. With so many people falling victim to this dreaded disease, it was very difficult to muster the necessary burial details. In desperation, the French government released four condemned convicts from prison and forced them to collect and bury the diseased and highly infectious corpses.

Incredibly, the four condemned thieves appeared to be magically immune to the plague in spite of their close contact with infected bodies in various stages of decay. When the plague had finally run its awful course, the four thieves were promised their freedom if they would reveal the "magic" they used to remain healthy when all around them were dying of the Black Death.

According to the legend, the "magic" potion the condemned men drank daily was a generous portion of sour wine—well steeped with fresh-crushed garlic cloves! This mixture has become known as "Vinaigre des Quatre Voleurs"—Four Thieves Vinegar—and is still sold in

France today!

Just what is this "magic" herb? The Encyclopedia Britannica tells us that garlic (Allium Sativum) is a bulbous perennial plant of the lily family and is used to flavor foods. The aroma is powerful and onion-like and the taste is pungent. Garlic is a classic ingredient of many national cuisines and has only become popular in the United States since World War II. The bulb contains an antibiotic, allicin. Garlic has antiseptic properties and is an expectorant and intestinal antispasmodic.

Garlic is a native vegetable of Central Asia, an area of the world which includes northwest India, Afghanistan and parts of the U.S.S.R. and it grows wild in Italy and southern France. Other vegetables native to the region are carrots, muskmelon, onions, peas, radishes and spinach. Garlic is also indigenous to the Mediterranean, along with artichokes, asparagus, cabbage, celery, chickory, chives, cress, endive, beets, leeks, lettuce, onions, parsley, parsnips, peas, rhubarb and turnips.

The membranous skin of the bulb encloses up to twenty edible bulblets called cloves. Flower stalks sometimes arise bearing tiny bulblets and blossoms without seeds. Garlic is grown as an annual crop by methods similar to those used in growing onions. Garlic contains about 0.1% essential oil.

Garlic may have arrived on American shores by a circuitous route, but it has a lot of enthusiastic fans. "The Garlic Capital of the World," Gilroy, California (pop. 22,000), annually hosts a fun-filled festival dedicated to garlic. In July of 1984, more than 150,000 garlic fanciers attended!

SCIENTIFIC STUDIES PROVE GARLIC A SUPERIOR NATURAL REMEDY

Science says both grandmother and the ancients were right. Among the traditional uses for garlic as a cure are such ailments as asthma, deafness, bronchial congestion, arteriosclerosis, fever, nightmares, circulatory problems and liver conditions. Today, science is not only substantiating the effectiveness of garlic as a remedy for these ills, but is uncovering more and more therapeutic uses for this odiferous herb as well.

Garlic protects against blood clots forming in the veins and its documented anti-clotting agents can help prevent heart attacks and strokes. American scientists have been successful in identifying a chemical, *ajoene,* in garlic which possesses amazing anti-clotting properties. Another chemical with the ability to inhibit the formation of potentially dangerous blood clots is *adenosine,* also present in garlic according to Dr. Martyn Bailey of George Washington University, Washington,D.C.

Garlic is both antiseptic and antibacterial. In fact, as long ago as 1858, Louis Pasteur, developer of the pasteurization process that protects our milk from bacterial contamination, reported on the antiseptic powers of garlic. Garlic shows anti-tumor activity and appears to have a tendency to inhibit malignant cells. Current research shows garlic, as a general fungicide, may actually improve the body's all-important immune responses.

Nutritionally speaking, a clove of garlic is an excellent source of potassium and phosphorus. It also contains significant amounts of Vitamins B and C, as well as calcium and protein. And garlic is rich in selenium, currently being studied as a possible heart-disease preventive itself. In addition, selenium is an antioxidant which is said to prevent the effects of aging. Selenium is probably 10 times stronger than Vitamin E and is especially effective in removing contamination by the heavy metals, such as lead and mercury, that enter our bodies through the food chain and the environmental pollution of the air and water supplies of much of the world.

In the laboratories of the world, medical researchers have found garlic to be an amazing natural remedy for many modern ills, including heart-disease, hypertension (high blood pressure), diabetes, dysentery, pneumonia, Candida Albicans (fungal/yeast infection) and many others. This wide-acting natural fungicide and antibiotic purifies the blood in the body, removes toxic substances from the cells (by chelation), improves the body's immune system, is a metabolic aid and helps keep weight levels down. Garlic encourages the secretion of hormones within the body, prevents fatigue, promotes the building of energy and helps retain vital B vitamins in the system.

HEALTH INSURANCE FOR THE HEART–In 1971, the University of Michigan mounted a study to discover if eating garlic's pungent oil in capsule form can reduce cholesterol levels in the body. Cholesterol is considered to be a major contributor to heart-disease when it builds up in fatty deposits on artery walls and reduces the flow of blood to the heart.

Two of the university researchers, Alan Tsai, Ph.D., and James Kelley, discovered that when rats were fed a diet moderately high in cholesterol, but which also included garlic, the cholesterol levels rose slightly, but stayed close to normal. Other rats fed the same diet, but without the addition of garlic, showed a sky-rocketing 23% increase in their cholesterol levels.

Dr. Hans Reuter, of Cologne, West Germany, found that garlic not only effectively controls cholesterol levels in the blood, but also removes toxins that interfere with the body's metabolism, including the fat-burning process.

Also in 1981, biochemist Amar Makheja, Ph.D., of the George Washington University School of Medicine in

Washington, D.C., studied garlic's ability to prevent blood clots and subsequent heart attacks. Dr. Makheja says, "The three active ingredients in garlic are adenosine, allicin and a sulphur compound. It's possible that the sulfur compound blocks thromboxane (a clotting agent) and that may be the reason garlic can prevent coronary thrombosis." Dr. Makheja says a regular consumption of garlic is necessary to continue the anticlotting effect in the blood.

A 1975 study published by Philadelphia's respected Wistar Institute of Anatomy and Biology showed that in rabbits fed a special diet designed to bring on atherosclerosis (hardening and clogging of the arteries), garlic oil reduced cholesterol levels by about 10%. Even better news was the fact that the average fatty deposit on the inner walls of the blood vessels was between 15% and an astounding 45% *less severe* in rabbits fed garlic oil.

These near-miraculous results were confirmed by the Department of Pathology of the R.N.T. Medical College in Udaipur, India where researchers found rabbits who received high cholesterol diets *with garlic oil* were protected to a significant extent. Their arteries were less pitted, showed less evidence of thickening and clogging, and their livers showed only a mild degree of fatty infiltration. Even more exciting was the fact that there was no evidence of cholesterol deposits in the hearts of the rabbits fed garlic oil.

Another Indian study, this time involving humans, was made at the Department of Pharmacology and Medicine, S.N. Medical College, Agra, India. Fed a diet especially prepared to elevate cholesterol levels, ten healthy volunteers ate a high-fat meal. After four hours, cholesterol levels were tested and found almost dangerously high. However, when the same high-fat meal was consumed with garlic, either raw or cooked, cholesterol levels stayed within the low-normal range.

THE CANCER CONNECTION—Wayne E. Criss,

Ph.D., of Howard's School of Human Ecology, Washington D.C., discovered in a series of experiments done in 1982 that cancers can't grow or spread without a substance called cyclic Guanosine Monophosphate, or cGMP. Dr. Criss then found that an extract from certain plants prevents the formation of cGMP in test tubes. The strongest source of this extract was—you guessed it—garlic!

An early study, published in 1957, continues to inspire scientists to study the effect of garlic on cancer. It was conducted at Case Western Reserve University in Cleveland, Ohio. The chief researcher thought rapidly dividing tissue, including cancer cells, required large amounts of sulfur amino acids. His idea was to cut down on -SH compounds to starve the cancer — and he suspected the active ingredient in garlic, *allicin,* would render the -SH harmless. He decided to find out in a hurry.

Could garlic prevent cancer in mice that had been injected with five million tumor cells that, under ordinary circumstances, would kill them within sixteen days? Producing allicin as nature does, the doctor crushed garlic cloves for his extract. He found that if the allicin was mixed with the tumor cells before the cells were placed in the mice, they didn't get cancer and they didn't die. Not after 16 days—and not after 6 months.

It was the promise shown by this study that encouraged a Japanese effort in 1964. Researchers Yanagi Kimura and Kotaro Yamamoto transplanted live cancer cells into a group of albino rats and injected them with a garlic extract four days later. Within only one hour, the extract produced a marked damage to the tumor cells by blocking the metaphase (a part of the rapid cell-division that characterizes cancer) and by preventing chromosomes from reproducing. Even twelve hours after injection, the garlic extract was still working, fighting about half of the tumor cells. The researchers reported that the tumors shrank, still a near-miraculous effect, but didn't disappear completely.

Three years later, two other Japanese scientists used garlic to develop a sort of "anti-cancer vaccine." As in the earlier American study, they found tumor cells mixed with garlic extract did not produce a cancer in mice. Carrying their experiments further, they found an injection of garlic-saturated tumor cells actually immunized the mice against at least one type of cancer.

The two researchers twice injected mice with their "anti-cancer vaccine" of live tumor cells soaked in garlic extract, giving the shots one week apart. When the mice were then injected with cancer cells fourteen days after immunization, none developed tumors and none died within a time period of 100 days when the experiment was ended. By comparison, mice injected with live tumor cells *without the vaccine* died within just 14 to 28 days.

Dr. Mei Xing of the Shandong Medical College believes his 1981 study of cancer rates in China shows that the regular consumption of garlic results in a lower rate of stomach cancer. Dr. Xing says garlic juice seems to inhibit the growth of bacteria in the stomach, with less formation of nitrites and nitrosamines. Nitrosamines are known to cause cancer in animals. In an experiment, he found that volunteers who took 1/3 ounce of homogenized fresh garlic reduced their nitrite levels significantly within only four hours. Dr. Xing says, "Garlic reduces the concentration of nitrite in the human stomach and may thus be considered as a protective factor against the development of gastric (stomach) cancer."

TRIPLE PROTECTION: ANTIBIOTIC, ANTIFUNGAL & BACTERIOSTATIC PROPERTIES—In testing antibiotics against various infections, clinical microbiologist Edward Delaha of Georgetown University Hospital of Washington, D.C. found garlic often works as well as chemically-manufactured antibiotics. Delaha says a shampoo of powdered garlic and chlorophyll might cure scalp infections, such as ringworm, and athlete's foot could be eliminated by a simple soaking in garlic water.

Delaha says, "Garlic seems to be extremely effective. They've been using injections of garlic extract on patients with a type of meningitis caused by a fungus in China. They've had an unbelievable cure rate, even with people who have been in comas."

YEAST INFECTIONS—The medical treatment of choice for fungal infections is the use of antifungal drugs. However, the side-effects of these prescribed drugs include the possibility of kidney damage, nausea, fever, skin rashes and so on. Science now recognizes that Candida Albicans, considered by many to be merely the vaginitis that plagues so many women, is actually a serious threat to health and can escalate into many more diseases, including meningitis and encephalitis. It is not limited to women only and typically attacks those in an already weakened condition from other illnesses.

Recent clinical research has identified Candida Albicans as the root cause of many symptoms, such as vaginitis (and a similar condition in the male partner), mouth thrush, tiredness, depression and even "bad moods." The symptoms of Candida can be manifested in anything from allergies and eye infections to an inflammation of the colon.

Fortunately, garlic is non-toxic and has been shown to inhibit the growth of fungus in the body without the adverse side-effects of drugs. The active component of garlic is stable in both the blood and stomach and acts effectively in the body's acidic environment.

The antibiotic, antifungal and bacteriostatic effects of garlic come from *allicin,* formed when the cellular membrane of the garlic clove is sliced or crushed. The cellular membrane separates an enzyme, *allinase,* and the substrate *alliin.* Mixed together, they create *allicin*—and the characteristic odor associated with this pungent herb. But it's the allicin we want. Allicin has the wonderful ability to attack harmful bacteria within the body without attacking and destroying the beneficial bacteria and digestive flora we need. In fact, some researchers have noted allicin can be more effective and is often needed in smaller quantities than penicillin.

Garlic has been called "Russian penicillin," probably because it was widely used by U.S.S.R. doctors to treat the wounded during two world wars. A cut clove of garlic was placed around infected wounds and held in place with a light bandage. Incredibly, within a few days, the wound was completely clean with no sign of infection or putrid flesh. Currently, U.S.S.R. scientists have discovered a method of reducing garlic to a vapor and this vapor is then inhaled. Unfortunately, I have been unable to turn up any concrete information as to the results of such a highly novel garlic treatment. It seems to me much easier just to add garlic to the daily diet in one form or another.

HIGH BLOOD PRESSURE—As long ago as 1948, a Dr. Piotrowski of the University of Geneva, publishing in the medical journal *PRAXIS,* reported on experiments he conducted with a group of 100 patients suffering from hypertension, or high blood pressure.

His research revealed that within three to five days of garlic treatment, over 40% of these patients had a satisfactory reduction in their blood pressure.

BLOOD SUGAR REDUCED IN DIABETICS—In a 1973 edition of *LANCET,* three doctors published reports showing that garlic was equally as effective as the drug *tolbutamide,* medical treatment of choice in the management of diabetes. The three doctors, working independently, all established that garlic, slower acting than the drug tolbutamide, could actually clear the blood stream of excessive glucose.

GARLIC AGAINST COLDS, COUGHS, BRONCHITIS, ASTHMA—A medical practitioner by the name of K. Nolfi, M.D., author of "My Experiences with Living

Food," writes that garlic is effective against all manner of respiratory infections. Dr. Nolfi's method of curing the common cold consists of holding a cut clove of garlic inside the mouth between the cheeks and teeth. It is said this method will cure a cold almost immediately. For more serious complaints, including badly inflamed tonsils and glands, laryngitis and bronchitis, the cut cloves of garlic must be renewed every few hours over a period of a few days. Dr. Nolfi also says a cut clove of garlic rubbed on the soles of the feet before retiring will often cure a cold overnight, but didn't explain how to avoid chasing your bed partner out of the room in the process!

As you can see from the studies reported on, the serious research on garlic's properties is currently centered on the effect this pungent herb has against the two biggest killers of modern times—cancer and heart-disease. Although the encouraging results being shown by scientists around the world are hard to believe in this chemically oriented and prescription drug age we live in, all are true and well-documented. This common herb, shunned by many sophisticated people because it causes "garlic-breath," has been proven of great value in over 5,000 years of recorded use, as well as in the laboratories of today.

MANY FORMS OF GARLIC ON THE MARKET

If you have decided to add garlic to your daily diet, as I have, you will probably want to visit a local health-food store and look over the many forms of garlic preparations currently on the market. When making your selection, make sure the product you select contains the natural *allicin,* the active antibiotic, antifungal and bacteriostatic component of raw garlic. Some manufacturers have taken out the allicin in order to produce an odorless garlic.

However, at least one responsible manufacturer, the Wakunaga Pharmaceutical Company of Japan, produces and distributes a deodorized garlic in tablets, capsules and liquid under the trademark *Kyolic*™. All Kyolic garlic products contain a modified form of allicin the company claims to be better than the real thing. As a chelating agent, Kyolic is said to exert a detoxifying effect which neutralizes heavy metal poisoning by binding with lead, mercury and cadmium and acts as an antioxidant as well, thus improving the function of the liver, kidneys, nervous system and circulatory system.

In addition to a liquid garlic extract, you will find other odorless forms still containing allicin, but specially processed to prevent any hint of garlic from tainting your breath. You might choose a garlic/parsley combination in either tablets or capsules, or even a potent 1000 mg garlic capsule with 2 mgs of nature's breath sweetener, chlorophyll.

If you decide on a capsule, I want to add one word of caution here, and this goes for any food product you purchase as well. *Be sure the product you choose is* not *made with* hydrogenated *oil of any type.* This is an all too-common ingredient in many processed foods. Doesn't sound threatening, does it? In fact, however, hydrogenated oil is extremely harmful to the body.

All natural fats and oils contain substances known as *antioxidants,* which prevent rancidity. When allowed to remain in foods, these *antioxidants prevent the destruction of Vitamins A, D, E, K, several B vitamins and carotene—not only in the food itself, but in the intestinal tract.* Without natural antioxidants, serious losses of these vitamins occur before they can reach the blood.

Unfortunately, the natural antioxidants are lost when fats and oils are hydrogenated. Hydrogen is added to the unfilled chain of essential fatty acids, destroying their health-building value. Untreated, unrefined cold-pressed oils still contain most of their antioxidants and can be purchased at most health-food stores.

Among the various forms of garlic available, my personal favorite remains the Garlic Pearles developed in 1920 by J.A. Hofels, a doctor then living in Great Britain. As a medical man and scientist, Dr. Hofels was well aware of what a wonderful food and medicine garlic is and mounted a very thorough and methodical study into the best way to prepare the herb for use as a daily supplement to the diet. Deciding it was vital to overcome the prejudice against the odor, Dr. Hofels discovered the ways and means of encapsulating all the essential vital oils from fresh garlic. Since digestion does not start until the potent capsule reaches the stomach, the breath remains sweet. From specially grown crops, Dr. Hofels produced Garlic Pearles, which have become a tremendous success and which are still used in many countries throughout the world today.

If you fancy fresh garlic, but don't want to offend others with the pungency of your breath, one recommended method is to finely mince a portion of a clove, put it in a teaspoon and place it on the back of your tongue. Swallow quickly with a glass of water. Chewing is what releases garlic's characteristic odor and causes it to scent—or foul—the breath, depending on your point of view!

One husband and wife I know of have solved the breath problem in still another way. Neither wishes to offend the other, but both believe very strongly in the health-promoting and preventive effects of fresh garlic. Here's what they do. Just before retiring, the wife chops a fresh-cut clove into small pieces. Then she peels a banana, slits it down the middle and tucks the garlic inside. Both husband and wife eat their half-banana laced with garlic and they go to bed. They report there is absolutely no odor of garlic on the breath, not even the next morning!

Whatever your choice, remember garlic is highly effective as a natural preventive and should be taken daily for best results.

Noel Johnson—86-Year Old Marathon Runner
What's his secret?

BEE POLLEN

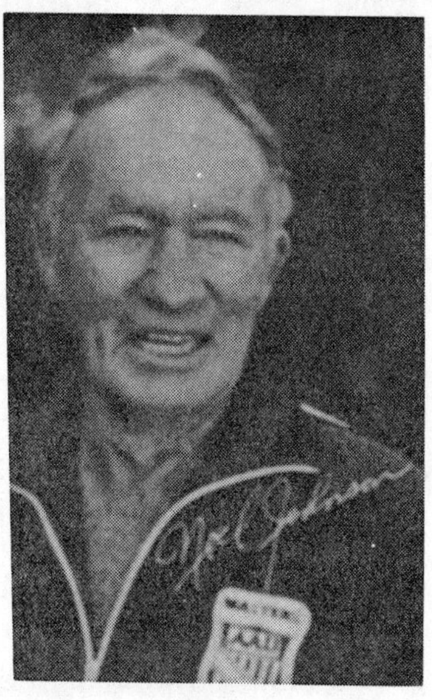

At 84 years of age, Noel Johnson was honored with the *President's Council on Physical Fitness & Sports Award.* The President's Council believes Johnson's healthy lifestyle is precisely the example millions of Americans need. Now 86, Noel competes in marathons around the world and has the gold medals to prove it. He holds the World's Senior Boxing Championship, often fighting men 30 years his junior to keep it. In 1984, he visited both Japan and Iceland lecturing, running and promoting his autobiography, which has been translated into both languages. In 1985, Noel Johnson applied to be the first octogenarian in space!

He has been recommended to NASA and just might end up being the world's oldest space cadet on some future space flight.

"I WANT THE BEST BEE POLLEN IN THE WORLD"

By B.R. Brown

I didn't know it back in 1975 when I told my staff, "I want the best bee pollen in the world," but these nine words launched a personal research project that developed into what is now the largest harvester, distributor, marketer and developer of beehive products in the United States, the C C Pollen Company. In brief, here's how it came about.

In the 1940s before America's entry into World War II, I joined the Royal Canadian Air Force as a fighter pilot. It was in London while I was flying with the British Royal Air Force that I was introduced to bee pollen in the officer's mess by a fellow pilot. His description of the benefits of these golden grains was over-enthusiastic, to say the least. As a matter of fact, he became something of a pest on the subject. I just couldn't believe such a simple little food could possibly be the miraculous substance he claimed it was and I promptly forgot all about it.

By the 1960s, I was back in the states, married and a father of two. I ran across some articles on bee pollen relating some interesting studies done abroad that seemed to bear out the truth of my friend's statements. I still wasn't convinced, but I decided to try it out for myself and began purchasing bee pollen tablets in a local health food store. They were hard and dry and not very tasty, but I insisted the whole family partake and it did seem we all stayed pretty healthy. I didn't know it at the time, but these tablets were made with Spanish bee pollen.

As I continued on with my health research, I learned those bee pollen tablets were from Spain and the tablets were made from a single pollen source, the Jara plant, and were old and not fresh. My research indicated I should find a bee pollen from many pollen sources as beehive-fresh as possible. My patriotism demanded I buy American.

I searched and found a California beekeeper who agreed to sell me a multi-colored pollen, proving it was from many pollen sources, which was frozen right out of the beehive to preserve beehive-freshness. He packaged it for me in 30 pound buckets and I probably purchased about 150 pounds per year for many years. What a difference! These fresh granules actually tasted good!

By the early 1970s, it became apparent that *something* was making a difference in our household. Both my children received awards for perfect attendance in school and not one of us was ever sick, not even with a sniffle or a bout with the flu. We didn't even have a family doctor because we had no need for one. I was convinced. It simply had to be the bee pollen and it was then that I determined to do some serious in-depth research on this product of the beehive.

At that time, I was in a partnership involved with the stock market, providing a highly successful and financially rewarding investment advisory service. But once I started ferreting out and reading the research and double-blind studies on the incredible potency of the little golden grains from the beehive, I was hooked. I lost interest in the stock market, sold the investment advisory service, dissolved the partnership and devoted myself full-time to the study of bee pollen.

It wasn't easy accumulating this material either. Much of the research on the products of the beehive was (and is still) conducted in the Soviet bloc countries. It took time, money, perseverance and determination to persuade them to provide us copies. And, once received, we still had to have them translated! Knowing what I know now about the miraculous benefits of this natural food, I'm very thankful I persisted.

Published studies from authorities around the world

confirmed that heat-treated pollen was robbed of many vital nutrients and the heat-treating destroyed vital enzyme action as well. This discovery led me to make two trips abroad to investigate foreign beekeeping methods and I was disturbed to find that most foreign pollens were, of necessity, heat-treated because they were harvested in humid climates and deep-freeze storage facilities were not available.

Further research revealed pollen loses up to 76% of its nutritive value during a year when dried and not stored frozen. Since foreign pollens cannot reach the American consumer much before they are 4 to 6 months old, I concluded this combination of aged pollen and heat-processed dried pollen was devastating to the quality. These were not the pollens I was seeking.

The decision to harvest *naturally-dry* high-desert Arizona Rocky Mountain pollen was prompted by research done by Dr. Nicolai Vasilievich Tsitsin, Chief Biologist of the U.S.S.R. Tsitsin discovered the 200 or more people documented over 125 years of age in Russia used pollen and honey collected in the *high, dry desert-like climate of the Caucasus Mountains* in upper Russia as their main source of nourishment. Dr. Tsitsin attributed their longevity to the action of the naturally dry pollen harvested from desert growth and concluded bee pollen taken regularly in sufficient amounts will prolong the life-span.

When equally well accredited scientists confirmed this premise, I was elated! The climate in my own state of Arizona met Tsitsin's requirements perfectly. Working with a Master Beekeeper, we began fitting beehives with pollen traps, C C Pollen Company was formed and High-Desert® Honeybee Pollen was born. It was sweet, fresh and delicious and I began to believe I had fulfilled my objective of finding the "best bee pollen in the world."

But when continuing research showed even my High-Desert® pollens harvested in some of the virgin Rocky

Mountain areas of Arizona were deficient in selenium, potassium and some other soil nutrients, I was devastated! What to do? I was searching for the most perfect bee pollen possible and still felt our Arizona High-Desert® bee pollen was the best bee pollen currently available on the world market—but I also realized even High-Desert® could be improved.

Three and a half years of intensive research lay ahead. Every Federal government source, every U.S. Agricultural Department source, every County Extension agent and every other source we could find was contacted to learn the soil deficiencies and soil excesses of all 48 states. This information was then laboriously consolidated and extensively analyzed.

We now know the general soil nutrient profile of each of the 48 states. For example, North and South Dakota, some parts of Colorado, New Mexico and Arizona have high concentrations of selenium in their soils. But the entire Northern areas of the U.S. once covered by glaciers, the East Coast, most of California, all of Oregon and the state of Washington have soils deficient in selenium, zinc, iodine and all other water-soluble nutrients.

It appeared the only way to deliver as near-perfect bee pollen as possible was to blend pollens from many areas. However, we really didn't want to go to the trouble and expense of mixing pollens from many areas. Why? Because it is a very costly procedure. We realized the blending process would result in an excessive powdering of the fragile granules and we would lose a high percentage.

Reluctantly, I concluded we could only hope to achieve "the only *perfect* bee pollen in the world" by mixing and blending pollens from many, many areas. It was absolutely vital we mix bee pollens from areas having a high concentration of certain soil nutrients and a low concentration of others with pollens from areas having the opposite percentages.

We were forced to start harvesting bee pollen from North and South Dakota, all the Rocky Mountain states and most of the Western states to achieve the mixture most desirable to provide that perfect bee pollen. Now, we often blend pollens from as many as 20 different states.

Our expanded range of pollen harvesting leads us to believe that *only* C C Pollen Company produces the unique blend of many, many pollens to insure highest potency and complete nutrient content. We now harvest and market High-Desert® Honeybee Pollen*S*™, the *"S"* signifying the all-important blend, beautifully trademarked as *"The Pollen of 10,000 Flowers"*. This single innovation alone makes High-Desert® preeminent in the field and puts all C C Pollen Company products clearly in a superior class by themselves, far ahead of any other bee pollen products currently on the world market.

We believe we are the only food producer in the world both aware of these documented soil deficiencies—and doing something about it. High-Desert® just might be the *only* nutritionally complete food available anywhere on this planet.

As a case in point, a recent study just received (translation from the German) entitled, "Bee Pollen—A Valuable Part of Holistic Therapy," states, "Being concerned about the widespread development of disease and the detrimental effects of modern civilization—often caused by our refined, beautified and mostly denatured foods, termed *mesothropy (semi-nutrition)*—it became clear we must seek the solution where nature still functions. Fortunately, the world of the bee is such a "bastion of nature." It's my guess that if soil samples were taken around the world wherever foods are grown, the results would show a great depletion of certain essential nutrients, exactly as the U.S. studies proved.

Incidentally, all High-Desert® products are preserved

with cold—not damaging heat. Fresh granules are frozen upon harvest by the beekeeper and held frozen until shipment to us. Once they are packaged, all products are held in deep-cold storage of -15 degrees F. until shipment to the purchaser, as extensive research dictates.

Today, I can honestly say I have actually achieved the goal I set for myself so many *costly* long years ago. *I am certain High-Desert® is the "best bee pollen in the world today."* My family eats it everyday. I eat it everyday and I know.

You wouldn't believe how the company and our research files have grown over the years. Quality creates its own market. In 1975, we started in a corner of my offices, with a staff of three, and C C Pollen Company now has many hundreds of beekeepers, in-house personnel today numbers 28 and occupies a suite of offices, plus we are computerized to enable us to do business around the world. High-Desert® apiaries (bee yards) are now established in many states besides Arizona. Most of the health-food stores in this country carry C C Pollen Company products, as well as do some supermarkets and pharmacies. We are international and market a heavy volume in many countries of the world.

As a matter of fact, if anyone asks you what President Ronald Reagan, Loni Anderson, Steve Riddick (said to be the fastest man in the world), Dr. Remy Chauvin (Director of the Paris Child Preventatorium), the original Greek Olympic athletes, some current Olympic gold medal winners—and Noel Johnson, the 86-year old marathon runner who contributed the following chapters on pollen—have in common, confidently answer *bee pollen.* Everyone mentioned above is a bee pollen fan.

In addition, ancient texts and religious writings the world over praise honeybee pollen as 'food of the gods' and agree this revered substance contains the secret of eternal youth, health and longevity. More and more consumers all over the world today are agreeing with that appraisal.

Am I satisfied? For the moment, yes. We do it right. But the research continues and who knows what advances science might make in the next decade? I promise you, if new research shows a better way to harvest, produce, process, handle or store beehive products, C C Pollen Company will be the first to know. And C C Pollen Company won't drag its feet about putting new ideas into production either, no matter what cash outlay is required. Remember, I eat it—and I have always demanded *"the best bee pollen in the world."*

NOEL JOHNSON
86-YEAR OLD SUPERMAN!

His Words—His Story

I was born in July of 1899, before the century turned. I was an enthusiastic part of the fabled Roaring 20s, the "flaming youth" of the time, and I enjoyed every minute of it.

When I finished school in 1921, I refused a job with the Great Northern Railway and hot-footed it home to Heron Lake, Minnesota and a snappy little red-head named Zola Mae Dalzell. We were married on the last day of 1921 and Zola joked I'd better never forget our anniversary.

After spending two years "down on the farm," we were restless and ready for some excitement. We bought a Model T Ford, the most reliable of all cars on the road, for $350 and decided to go cross country to the State of Washington where Zola's cousins lived. It was autumn and the frosty air had a zing to it already and we were itching to get going.

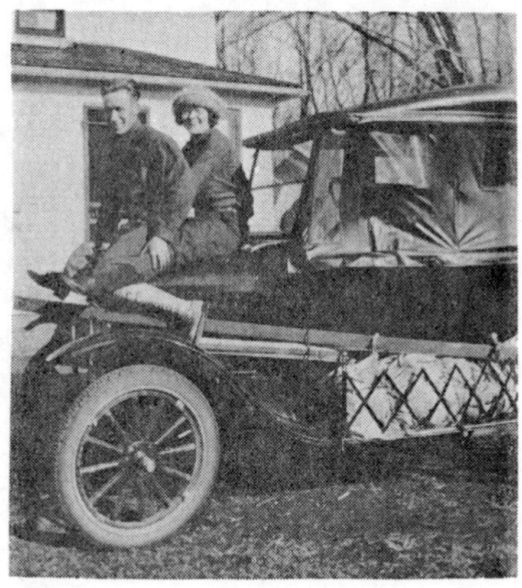

November, 1923. Packed and ready to leave.

Our shiny new car was elegantly equipped with side curtains, running boards and folding top. We had the front seats altered so they would recline, making it comfortable to sleep in the car. We fixed up a place above the back seat for groceries and bought a Coleman stove for cooking and heat. We purchased a tent big enough to cover the entire car to protect us on our stop-overs from snow, rain and wind.

With three spare tires on the back of the car, full water, gas and oil cans strapped on the running boards, plus heavy winter clothing, blankets and bedding packed, we were ready to start out in what was probably the first "camper" on the road anywhere.

Back in 1923, it was common for folks to travel in "caravans" of several cars for safety and as a precaution against being stranded in some muddy ditch. Few roads were well-traveled and you couldn't count on help being available when it was needed. Back then, garages and gas stations were few and far between and the quality of your driving wasn't nearly as important as your skill as a mechanic!

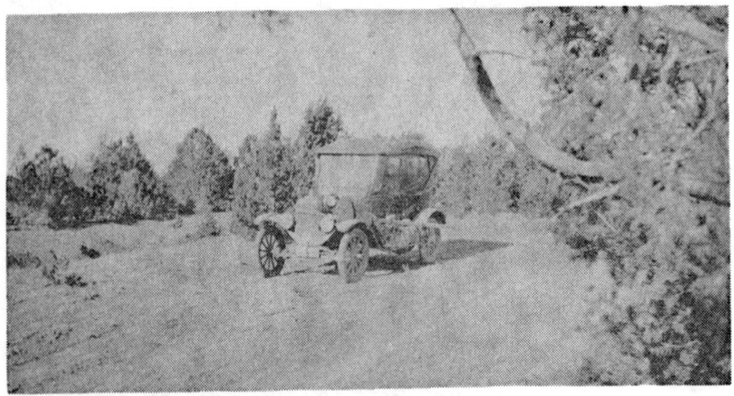

Entering California in January, 1924.

Our parents were worried, but we set out the last week of November 1923, chasing the sun south. We finally made it to California in January of 1924 after being on the road for over five weeks, eating, sleeping and living in the car the entire time. The shine was off the Ford by the time we reached California, but we were soaking up the sun and ready to take on the world. We forgot about going on to Washington State and settled in.

After a successful athletic career in college, I continued on with my boxing on the side and got a regular job with Convair Industries as well. The hospitable Californians gathered us in and soon we were embarked on a round of parties and cookouts on the beach. It was all great fun and we ate and drank with the best of 'em. Even the birth of our two children didn't slow us down much and we figured life couldn't get much better than this. Pretty ordinary stuff, right?

I sure didn't know it then, but this free and easy lifestyle was the largest contributing factor to my early decline into dangerously poor health. When I retired at 65, my Zola was in a nursing home with a stroke that left her comatose. My only physical activity was visiting Zola daily, hoping in vain she would open her eyes and flash her old mischievous smile at me. I shuffled around the house, drank a lot of beer and ate whatever came to hand, mostly manufactured junk-food.

By the time I was 70, I had faced the fact that my Zola was lost to me forever. The only joy I had in my life seemed to be my great-grandsons, but even the close relationship I had with my son and daughter and their families wasn't enough to bring me out of my deep funk.

My doctor had diagnosed me as having a serious heart condition and restricted my physical activity. He told me I didn't even dare mow the lawn, saying I might not live to trim the borders. It sure was easy to follow his orders. I just didn't much care about anything. I realize now I was simply waiting for the next and final stop on the journey we call life. I considered I had lived my Biblical three-score years and ten. In the traditional and conventional sense, my life was over. *Or was it?*

I was worrying my family, living alone and sinking fast, eating improperly and deteriorating daily. My son, Jim, voiced his concern with affection and proposed that I go to the hospital for a complete and thorough checkup. It was becoming apparent, he said, I would soon need someone to look after me.

He was right. I certainly wasn't doing a good job of looking after myself. By then I was 40 pounds overweight, putting a strain on my already damaged heart, and couldn't function well.

The next morning I looked in the mirror and realized I looked and felt like an old man. For the first 70 years of my life, I had "followed the pattern" and lived like everyone else, did what everyone else did. The condition I found myself in at 70 years of age was no different than unnumbered others before me. It's "normal" to be ill and aging at 70. After all, this is merely the natural progression of events. *Or is it?*

I finally did something I had been carefully avoiding for a long time. I thought—*hard.* I was very clear on what I *didn't* want. I didn't want to be a burden to my children. I didn't want to be bedridden and helpless. I felt it was still my responsibility to take charge of my own life and health. I didn't want to turn that responsibility over to anyone else.

I stripped down and looked in the mirror. All the classic signs of aging and ill-health were there. I was overweight, with a bulging gut, lackluster eyes, unused muscles hanging slack.

I looked defeated. But I used to be a fighter and the thought "defeated" stirred something in my ego. Here I was, about to give up and take the count. I decided then and there to beat the bell and come out swinging. They can't count you out when you're trying.

One of the announcers hung the name "Battling Blue Eyes" on me in my early years as a boxer. Well, I had the battle of my life ahead of me to get back in condition, but I was determined to do it. "Battling Blue Eyes" was back!

And I succeeded. Sure, it took awhile, but with a program of good nutrition, with bee pollen my secret weapon, a gradually escalating program of exercise and determination, *I made it . . . and you can, too.*

One of the highlights of my "second lifetime," occurred in 1976. I was tickled pink to be approached by the *Wheaties* people. They asked permission to feature me on the Wheaties box as part of their *Breakfast of Champions* series. It was a real kick to find myself in stores all over the world on five million boxes of Wheaties in 1977.

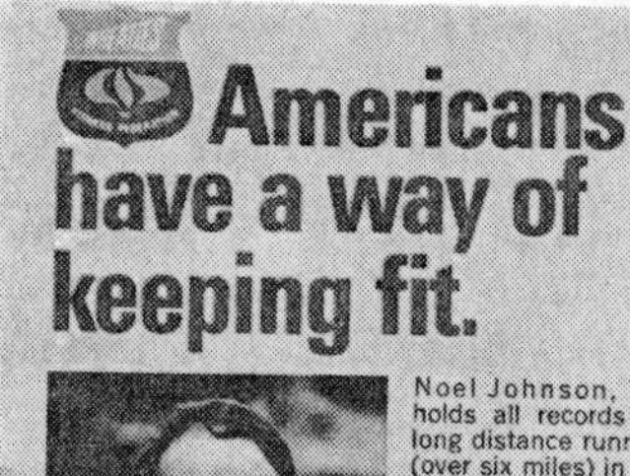

Americans have a way of keeping fit.

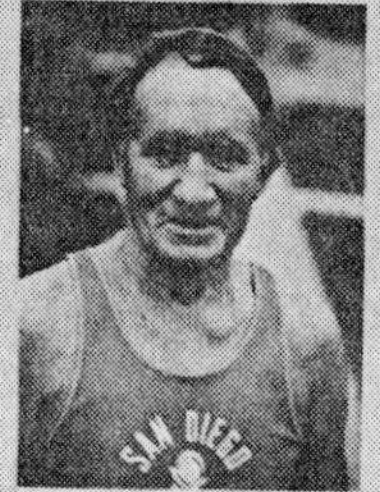

Noel Johnson, 76, holds all records for long distance running (over six miles) in the 70-75 age bracket of the AAU Masters Program. He is the only one in the world his age who runs the 26-mile marathon.

Noel is a member of the "Life Begins at 60" group. In 1974, the group ran a 300-mile relay from Hollywood to Las Vegas in 40 hours and 30 minutes (which certainly shows that people of all ages can remain physically fit).

"Jogging is the best thing I can do for my body. It gets my blood circulating, keeps my heart strong and increases my wind and endurance. I never have to worry about stiffness, arthritis or muscle strain. I have one special exercise I do for stretching my arms, legs, neck and spine. I stand erect, hold my arms out horizontally and twist my upper torso and arms to the right as far as possible. At the same time I kick my right leg in the opposite direction (left). I straighten out and repeat the exercise on the other side.

"Another reason I am so healthy is because I eat well. It's important to eat good, nutritional food."

Noel started his fitness program at 70. "When I started out, I couldn't make it a quarter of a mile around the high school track. I walked part, ran part, until I finally built myself up to where I could run a quarter of a mile. If you set your mind to it, anyone at any age can get himself in good physical shape. It's never too late but you can't do it overnight."

If you are over 40 or have a known health problem, consult your physician before beginning a physical fitness program.

Win the Presidential Sports Award in Your Favorite Sport.

The President's Council on Physical Fitness and Sports offers you the Presidential Sports Award in 39 different sports. For information on how to achieve the award in your sport, write: The Presidential Sports Award, P.O. Box 14, Greene, Rhode Island 02827.

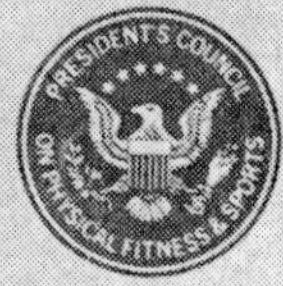

(The above does not constitute endorsement of product.)

Five Million Wheaties "Breakfast of Champions" boxes carried my picture and brief profile in 1977.

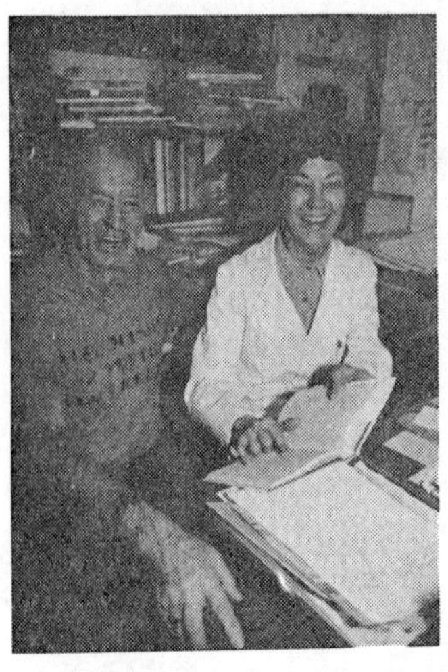

Today, at 86 years of age, the doctors who have examined me trying to find out how I've reversed the aging process, call me "superman."

At left, with Dr. Lenora Zohman, a respected cardiologist. Dr. Zohman is explaining the forthcoming tests to me.

Wired for 24 hours. A tape was running constantly and recorded all my vital signs.

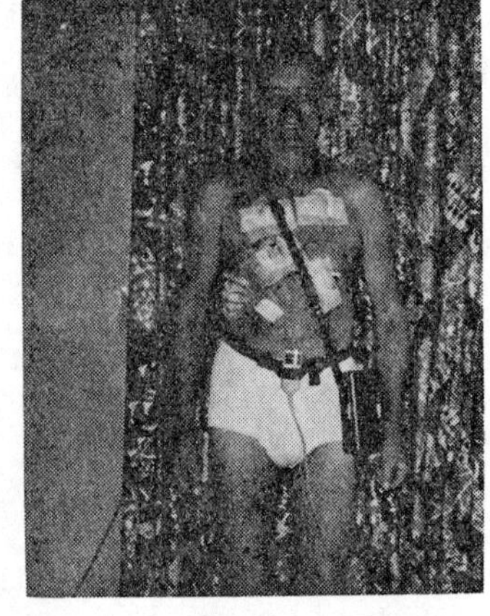

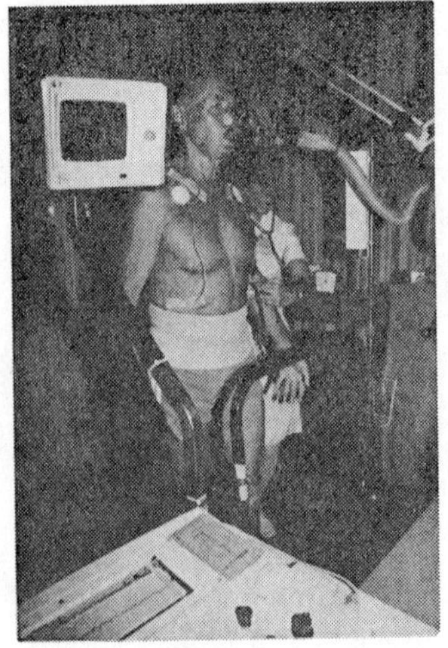

Breathing hard. Measuring lung capacity.

I've been on many television shows, including *To Tell the Truth, The Price is Right, The Richard Simmons Show, Dan Rather's Evening News,* and *David Letterman's late show.* Imagine being considered a celebrity just because you can still function in your 70s and 80s!

When I appeared on the *Tom Snyder Show* in Los Angeles in 1973, a doctor specializing in geriatrics was there to debate with me. The doctor seemed to think it was "normal" to have what he called "old-age" diseases after 65 or 70 years of age. He said "everyone did." I told him I was sorry *he* wouldn't live long enough to find out I wasn't "normal," as I would never have the "old-age" diseases he was talking about. Now, 13 years later, I'm still as healthy as a horse. I wonder how *he's* doing today.

I hold the title of "World's Senior Boxing Championship," and have issued a statement I will take on any challengers in my weight class over the age of 40. If they're over 60, I'll go easy on 'em.

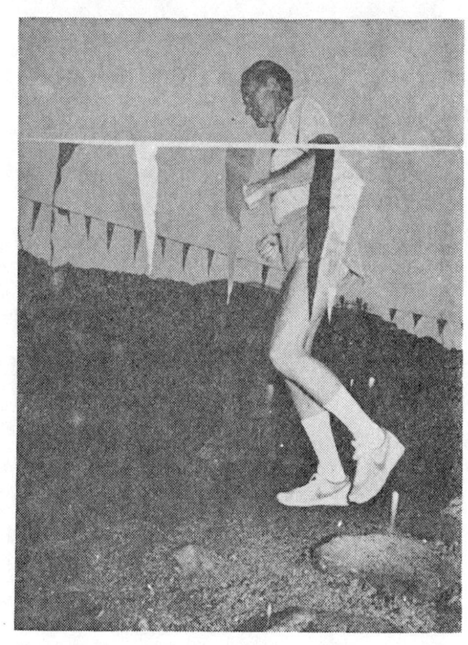

I run marathons of 26+ miles around the world, including Pike's Peak (straight *up* over 14,000 feet), and have the gold medals to prove it!

Crossing the finish line of the Pike's Peak Marathon

In 1984, I received the "Presidential Fitness Award;" I gave some talks and ran some races in both Japan and Iceland; my book, *A Dud at 70—A Stud at 80,* has been translated into Japanese and Icelandic and the peoples of those countries seem to have taken me to their hearts. I ran the New York Marathon for the fourth time in October of 1984 and I'm proud to be able to say I've bettered my time every year. In fact, I came home to California and ran another marathon for good measure! Best of all, I enjoy dining, dancing and romancing the ladies again!

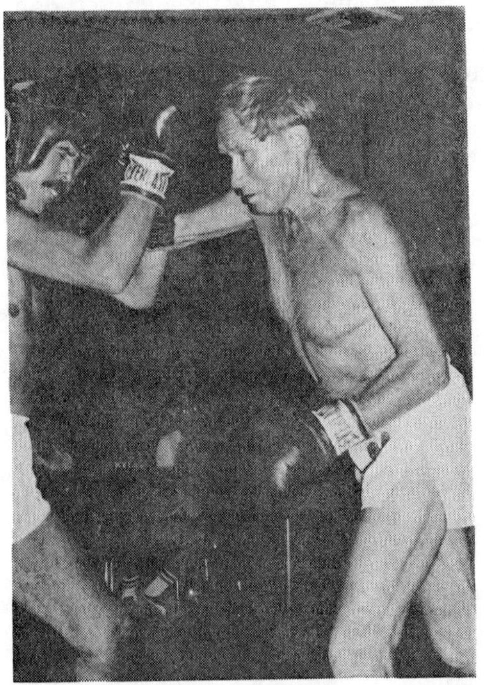

"Why can't an 80-year old man fight a 20-year old in the same weight class? I want to show that a man of 80 can be as good as the kids of 20," says Johnson.

Last July he won his fifth straight title in the 10th annual Senior Olympics Boxing Championship in Los Angeles, defeating his 40-year old opponent.

My fight with Leo Pereira in 1979. He was 40 and I was 80.

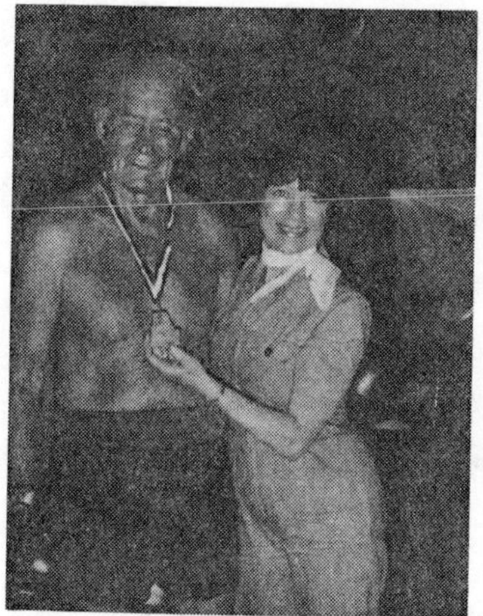

Sybil Jason presenting me with the gold medal after the fight.

Who wouldn't enjoy dancing with these pretty gals? My partner in the ballroom is Fern and Doreen is my square-dance partner and makes our outfits herself. Two very talented and lovely ladies.

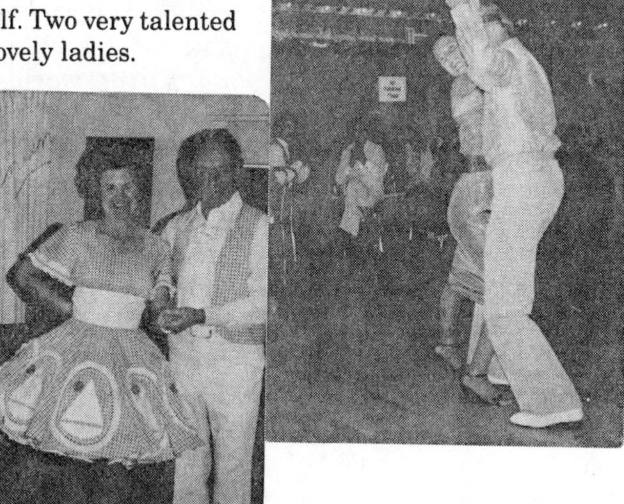

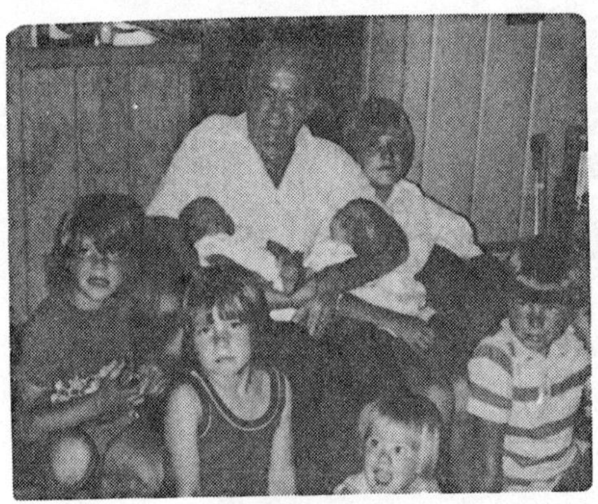

My 7 handsome great-grandsons. You better believe I'm proud of these boys!

What's next? Remember the song, "Fly Me to the Moon?" I want to be the first octogenarian in space. Can I do it? You bet! I *know* I can do it, but it now remains to convince NASA I'd be an asset as the world's oldest space cadet. Senator Pete Wilson has sent NASA my name and told them, "If you need an 86-year old who can run marathons, Noel Johnson is the perfect candidate."

Keep your eye on me—you ain't seen nothin' yet! I'm just rarin' to go. I feel good. I'm excited about the future and, after doing *A Dud at 70—A Stud at 80* in 1982, I'm looking forward to doing another book, *Living & Loving in my Third Century,* in the year 2000 when I'll be 101 years old. Now that's confidence!

To sum it all up, I know I'll be in better condition at 90 than I am today at 86 because I know what you have to do to rebuild and keep your cells alive and I know what causes illness! *Read on, and let me introduce you to "Pollen Power!"*

IMPOTENCE–CAUSE & EFFECT

Analysis of the Condition & What Cured Me

I'm gonna change my way of livin',
And if that ain't enough,
I'm gonna change the way I strut my stuff!
Nobody wants you when you're old and gray
They'll be some changes made today
They'll be some changes made!

. . . Old Song

Sexual problems can be classified simply as either physical or mental in origin. A surprisingly large number of people experience, at varying times in life, sexual problems that are actually by-products of other conditions. Anything that interferes with normal body functioning can cause some degree of trouble.

Further, we are conditioned to believe the sexual myth that good, mature sex must include rapid erection, extended foreplay, long drawn-out penetration and, finally, simultaneous orgasm. Sex manuals, marriage books, movies and even magazines continually reinforce this as the ideal. Unfortunately, these demanding conditions cannot always be met, bringing on feelings of inadequacy, guilt and anxiety.

I know from personal experience that most of the blame is placed on the man when he can't perform as expected. There is much written today about the increasing number of men, both young and old, who are impotent. What I've read and heard about the generally poor physical condition of both young and old, men and women, is not conducive to making love, but at least it confirms that it's not always the man's fault. At one time I too thought it was, but I now believe the ladies bear at least 50% responsibility for this phenomenon.

No matter how potent the man is, if the lady's not in

the mood—and won't cooperate to get in the mood—this will take the starch out of a man quick as anything. If the lady has the proverbial headache, the act may be satisfactorily consummated, but without any real satisfaction for either party. This sets the stage for a less pleasurable "next time."

In many East Asian countries, love-making is a craft to be practiced to perfection. Women are trained in this art and eagerly take their share of the responsibility as an equal partner in the love-pleasure experience. The Oriental culture teaches the sexual experience as something to be lovingly revered and enjoyed, while many of us are still struggling with 18th century Victorian moralities.

I believe many so-called impotent men would not be impotent if they had the cooperation they need. Even a potent man needs a willing, stimulating and participating partner who wants to make love. It does take two to tango. You can't dance if you're supporting or dragging an unenthusiastic, unwilling partner around the ballroom. It takes mutual cooperation to enjoy this graceful and sensuous dance.

The Encyclopedia Britannica defines both frigidity (women) and impotence (men) in the same paragraph as: "The incapacity to achieve full sexual satisfaction.

"The causes of frigidity may be organic or psychological. Any organic cause, anatomical or hormonal abnormality may result in painful intercourse or the inability to become aroused sexually. Clinicians universally agree that most frigid women are psychologically inhibited by guilt, shame, distress or a strained relationship with the sex partner.

"Male impotence, or incapacity to have normal coitus, may involve either an inability to maintain a satisfactory penile erection or an anatomical deficiency. Partial impotence refers to premature ejaculation of the seminal fluid, either before penetration of the woman or immediately thereafter."

Impotence may be caused by lower than normal functioning of the testes, by hardening of the arteries or by an abnormal condition of the nervous system. Certain prescribed medications for the treatment of peptic ulcer, high blood pressure or psychiatric conditions can also adversely affect sexual ability.

The foremost contributory factor in impotence is poor physical condition. A chronic low-grade barely detectable infection, resulting in fatigue and apathy, is more common than generally supposed. Lack of sufficient exercise and an inadequate diet keep much of the population teetering between poor health and real illness. There are far too many men and women who consider themselves well-fed, but who are in reality so poorly nourished and in such poor physical condition that they have no interest in making love.

In a recent well-publicized article, it was announced that a great discovery had been made by some brilliant men. They found a greater percentage of impotence among men suffering from diabetes. Diabetes, of course, is a *metabolic* disease in which there is either inadequate secretion of insulin or an inability of the body to utilize efficiently the insulin produced. (Bee pollen may correct a metabolic imbalance.) Their conclusion was that perhaps diabetes had something to do with being impotent. This thinking is incredibly simplistic. Diabetes or no diabetes, if you are ill for any reason, it will affect your body in every way—physically, mentally and sexually. When you correct your health, you obviously improve your performance in bed along with everything else.

The condition of the body is all-important. If you are not in as good physical condition today as you were a year ago, or five years ago, think what you will be like in future years. It's been said that before age 40, health pursues you, but after age 40, you must pursue health.

Now is the time to make the change. If proper methods are used, it won't take long to change from illness to health. It's never too late to start. Remember that I was 70 years old before I discovered the secrets that changed me from illness to health—from an old worn-out dud into a vital and energized stud.

The true foundation for my seemingly miraculous return to full-manhood began with my discovery of bee pollen. Bee pollen contains a gonadatropic hormone, a plant hormone similar to the pituitary sex hormone, gonadatropin, which functions as a sex gland stimulant. The results of bee pollen on impotence have been well documented by a study conducted at the University of Sarajevo in Yugoslavia with a group of men who could not satisfactorily have sexual intercourse and who had a low sperm count. After just one month of taking bee pollen, over half showed an improvement in sperm production, in better sexual performance and exhibited regained self-confidence as well. The complete story on bee pollen and its documented benefits are treated in a separate chapter.

It's obvious that the proper feeding of the endocrine gland system, which includes the sex glands, is an absolute necessity for proper functioning. The effects of gland-malnutrition, incredibly widespread but not easily identified, is creating a nation of underfunctioning individuals. The hormonal secretions of your sex glands are directly responsible for fertility, drive, libido and ability to function. You must feed them correctly.

In the early days of the 20th century, the majority of the population enjoyed good natural food, although they didn't necessarily eat the so-called "balanced meals" the scientists of today advocate. It is apparent to me that since chemical additives have become commonplace, with growth-hormones being fed to meat animals, plus insecticides and chemical fertilizers used to grow more and more inferior crops—quantity at the expense of quality—that dangerous levels of these artificial substances have infiltrated our food chain to an alarming degree. Add to this the fact that many vitamins, minerals and important nutrients are inevitably lost in the processing of the food we put on our family table, and then put back in with artificial chemical compounds, loaded with preservatives, stabilizers and synthetic vitamins and minerals. It's no wonder the U.S. is declining yearly on the list of the world's healthiest countries. We are eating chemically processed, unnatural dead food and still we wonder why we have millions and millions of sick and unhealthy people in the richest country in the world.

By 1970, over 90% of our meat cattle and poultry were injected with artificial hormones or fed chemicals in their food. The effect of these synthetic hormones on the human male was dramatically demonstrated in an Italian resort area. The Italian studs found they were uniformly becoming impotent and evidencing disturbing female characteristics. Their beards stopped growing and their breasts were enlarging and becoming defined. Even visitors in the area were affected. Fortunately, a visiting doctor discovered an only partially dissolved hormone pellet in the grilled chicken he was served for dinner. The chicken for this popular dish was supplied by a local poultry farm. They had increased the productivity of their birds by implanting pellets of stilbestrol (synthetic estrogen, a female sex hormone). This brought the birds to market size in five months, instead of the usual eight. Quick profit was the motive, of course. The supplier was unconcerned about the effect this medicated meat had on the consumer.

Nature provides all life forms with a strong urge to propagate the species. Although hampered by pollution in the soil, water and air, plus man-made chemicals, plants continue to grow in the natural order, but are now of inferior quality. Many animals, fish and fowl have become extinct or put on the endangered species list due to man's manipulation of the environment. If we continue to accept additive-laden foods, water treated with powerful chemicals to purify it and make it safe for drinking, meat animals given hormones for fast growth to gain the fast buck, how long will it be before the human race is officially declared an endangered species? Our urge and ability to propagate and reproduce is diminishing by a measurable amount.

Sex glands need a continuing supply of specific nutrients to function normally. Vitamins, minerals, hormones, enzymes, coenzymes and natural mineral trace elements are vital to the health of the sexual reproductive system. Proper natural nutrition will maintain effective and trouble-free sexual function for life. That powerhouse of nutrients, bee pollen, contains them all, and affords protection against chemical additives and environmental poisons.

I believe the foods needed to condition the body for sex are different than the foods needed for other physical activities. A football player, for instance, uses a tremendous amount of pure brute strength in the course of a game. He needs muscle-building protein and energy-producing carbohydrates in large amounts. I call these foods "outside" foods because they are necessary for the "outside" of the body.

"Inside" foods, on the other hand, nourish the cells and organs of the body and are the live foods that produce and/or reproduce life, to my way of thinking. Bee pollen, the complete nutrient, is absolutely essential in nature to fertilize and reproduce so many different plants and species. It's at the top of the list. Live seeds of any kind that will germinate and thus reproduce themselves are next.

I eat a lot of the smaller seeds, like poppy seeds, sesame seeds, chia seeds, flax seeds, sunflower seeds, radish seeds and pumpkin seeds. You can eat dozens and dozens of these smaller seeds with all their variety of life-producing elements.

Beside the "inside" foods you need for a healthy reproductive system, I believe it's vitally important to have good blood circulation. One good way to accomplish this is by a regular running program. I recently read an article reporting on a questionnaire sent to thousands of men and women asking what they thought about how running affected their sex life. They wanted to determine if runners were better lovers.

Of course runners are better lovers! The article didn't say why and I don't think they know. Runners not only have improved blood circulation, but also benefit by the exercise they get in the leg, hip and genital area, just exactly where it's needed. There's never just one way to accomplish anything and other means of improving circulation in the genital area include massage techniques, certainly the most fun, alternate hot and cold compress applications, plus many other exercises besides running.

It is interesting to note the one food that appears more often than any other in ancient lore as an aphrodisiac is honey. When modern science has attempted to analyze these claims with the common honey of today that has been heated, strained, clarified and, in some cases, adulterated with glucose, they were found to be false. It is important to note that the original aphrodisiac was natural, raw honey loaded with bee pollen particles. It is the microscopic pollen dust suspended in raw honey that gives it a cloudy appearance. An analysis of bee pollen shows that it is the world's only complete food and contains *all* nutrients needed by mankind. It seems safe to conclude that the active ingredient in honey is, in fact, bee pollen.

Halvah is a popular ancient rejuvenator that has survived to this day, virtually unchanged, in the middle and far-eastern countries of the world. It is a mixture of ground sesame seed and raw honey and can be found in some health-food stores and the old-type farmer's markets in parts of the United States. You can easily make your own, if you like. Grind at least a cup of sesame seed and add honey until you have the consistency of a hard dough. Form into balls or cakes. Halvah cakes were reportedly carried by Roman legions as marching rations and a man was thought able to survive longer on Halvah than any other food of equal weight. Just make sure you use raw honey containing abundant bee pollen.

This nutritious combination provides abundant magnesium, potassium, lecithin, phosphorus and aspartic acid along with all other nutrients. Some doctors today prescribe a similar formula for the treatment of fatigue, insomnia and disinterest in lovemaking. Over 85% of those so treated have responded well and report a renewed zest for life and love.

You will find a sound nutritional program based on pure, natural and complete foods that supply all nutrients the body, including the sexual and reproductive system, requires—plus a lean, fit body conditioned by regular exercise—to be a most potent aphrodisiac, but a willing and enthusiastic partner is the most potent aphrodisiac of all.

The recipe for an intimate and deeply satisfying—both mentally and physically—love-making experience begins with the proper ingredients.

First, the desire, then a willing and participating object of your desire, plus two well-nourished and conditioned bodies that have the ability to respond to mutual mental and physical stimulation.

Mix gently and tenderly. Shake well and enjoy as often as you like.

POLLEN POWER

The Documented Benefits of Bee Pollen

"Let Your Food Be Your Medicine . . .
Let Your Medicine Be Your Food"
. . . Hippocrates

I have made honeybee pollen the one unvarying and essential foundation of my rejuvenation program. Since I discovered honeybee pollen at the age of 70, this perfect live food has restored my manhood, brought me to full vigor and sexual potency, and continues to nourish every cell in my body, while also protecting my health. I am simply never sick.

This incredible storehouse of vitamins, minerals, enzymes, coenzymes, hormones, amino acids (protein) and trace elements is nutritionally complete and has been proven by chemical analysis to be the only food on this sweet earth that contains every nutrient needed by mankind. The extraordinary richness and potency of bee pollen produces the energy I need for the marathons I have participated in in the past and still continue to run at age 86, plus other physical activities requiring stamina and strength.

I have not one doubt that honeybee pollen is the one perfect food known in the world today. I just can't overemphasize the amazing youthful health and vitality this living substance has brought into my life—and can bring to yours.

Bee pollen is not only the most potent and richest food in nature, its composition is unequalled by any other food. It is a pure, live vegetable source of all nutrients and is actually richer in protein than any animal source. Bee pollen contains an incredible 5 to 7 times more amino acids (protein) than meat, cheese or eggs of equal weight, plus all other nutrients in abundance.

According to "Liebig's Minimum Law," any element conveyed to the body must be complete and has a prescribed relationship to every other. All nutrients must be present before they can be effectively used by the body. The body uses the protein (or any other element) better if the selection of amino acids (or any other element) is large. Pollen contains approximately 25% protein of the type indispensable in the diet, the amino acids the body is not capable of manufacturing or synthesizing. Such a complete selection of the necessary amino acids is not found anywhere but in bee pollen. It is particularly concentrated in all nutrients necessary for life and contains many elements products of animal origin do not possess.

Where do we get this wonderful stuff? Pollen is collected by that miracle worker, the honeybee.

Bees live and work in colonies and are among the most industrious of the social insects. They are almost single-handedly responsible for the pollination of many agriculture crops, garden and wild flowers, trees, shrubs and other growth. Without the pollen-carrying honeybee, many species of plants would not otherwise be fertilized and would die out and become extinct.

The social organization of the bee colony is most evident in the division of labor. The work of the bee is determined by age and all tasks are performed in turn by the female worker bees.

The bee's first duty at one day of age is housekeeping and she begins by tidying up the nursery. The wax cells are cleaned, the waste matter removed, and the cells are lined with a disinfectant solution of bee propolis ready for the queen's deposit of eggs.

The queen is truly the Queen-Mother and is the only egg-layer in the hive. She is larger than the workers and drones (male bees) and is fed royal jelly and tended by her daughters the whole of her life. Her only function is to lay brood.

About three days after emergence as an adult worker,

the bee advances to brood nursing and provides the older larvae, still in the waxen cells, with honey and pollen. In her sixth day of life, she nurses the larvae with food secreted by the pharyngeal glands located in the top of her head.

After another ten days, at slightly over two-weeks old, the worker bee becomes a builder. She now secretes wax flakes from a gland in her abdomen and uses the wax to make the comb or repair any breaks. Soon after, she makes her first flight outside the hive.

On about her twentieth day, she begins guard duty and protects the entrance to the hive. By now both her pharyngeal and wax glands have degenerated. She will no longer need them.

Finally, she becomes a collector, a forager for food, and remains at this job for the rest of her life.

Pollen is the live male element of the flower and is necessary for fertilization of the species. It consists of 50/1000ths of a millimeter corpuscles and is formed at the free end of the stamen as a golden dust, an almost microscopic powder. This is where the bees forage and collect the pollen.

The bee has excellent equipment for her task. The enlarged and broadened tarsal segments of her back legs have a thick trimming of bristles called "pollen combs." The outside of the tibia is surrounded by a fringe of long hairs that enclose a smooth, slightly concave area called the "pollen basket" in which the pollen is carried home to the colony.

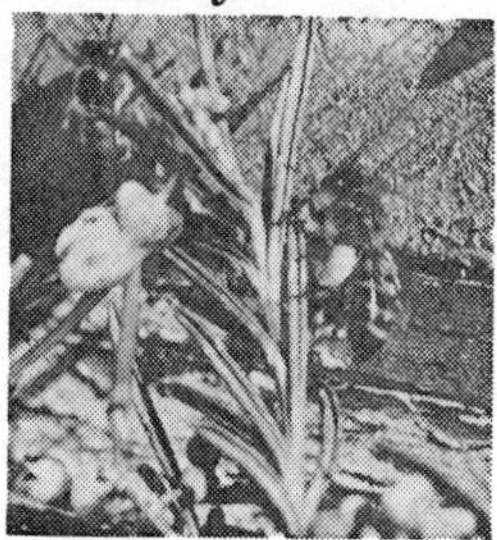

Inset shows a large kernel of pollen in the pollen-basket. This bee has visited approximately 1,500 flowers gathering the pollen for this one kernel.

Every worker bee fills her honey-sac on her way out of the hive. Once she selects a flower, she settles herself and scrapes the loose live pollen from the stamen with her jaws and front legs, moistening it with honey. As she flies on to the next blossom, she is feverishly moving her legs beneath her body. With her pollen combs, she scrapes the golden dust from her coat and legs, pressing it into her basket. As one lot after another, moistened with honey, is pushed into the basket, it gradually forms into a single grain. A bee must visit 1,500 flowers to fill her basket and a single golden grain contains upward of 500,000 to 5,000,000 live spores.

When she arrives home, she slips off the pollen kernel and deposits it in the wax comb. Pollen is sometimes called "bee bread" and is a necessary part of the bee's diet. Pollen and honey are stored in separate groups of cells inside the honeycomb to be used as needed. Although these two foods are not mixed together by the bee, raw honey in the comb is rich with pollen particles and bears little resemblance to the honey you find in your grocery store.

In order to harvest a portion of this live and potent life-giving substance for ourselves, a pollen trap is placed on the hive. This device consists of a box the same size as the man-made bee-box, or hive, and is equipped with a series of scientifically designed screens through which the bees pass to gain entrance to the colony. As they pass through the screens, approximately 60% of the pollen is gently brushed out of the pollen basket and falls through into the pollen drawer beneath.

The technology of the pollen trap is all-important. The trap must allow sufficient pollen through the screens for the feeding and maintenance of the colony and must allow the harvesting of the driest, cleanest pollen possible.

Moisture laden wet pollen from low-lying humid areas ferments quickly or molds and must be heat-treated

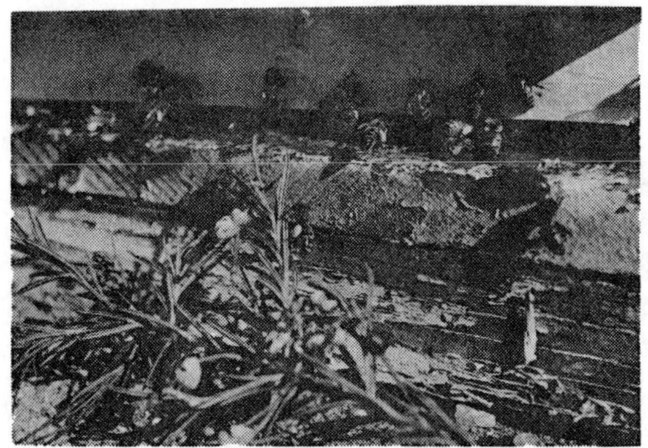

Pollen-laden honeybee bees entering the hive bringing food for the colony and for us.

immediately to preserve it for use. Heat processing kills the enzymes and reduces the nutrient value considerably, transforming the pollen into a dead food.

The solution to this dilemma is obvious. Honeybee pollen harvested in the high desert areas of the southwest United States comes naturally dry from the hive and requires no artificial heat processing. Because pollen improperly stored and handled loses up to 76% of its nutritive value in a year's space of time, the only satisfactory method of preserving fresh, live pollen is flash-freezing at zero degrees to maintain hive freshness indefinitely and preserve all the vitamins, minerals and other nutrients intact.

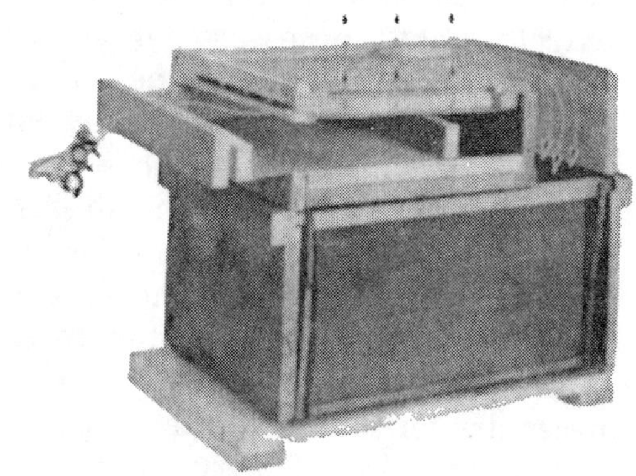

Cut away view of THE UNIVERSAL SUPER TRAP in the middle position showing the passage way of the bees, with the pollen drawer open and the top portion of the hive removed.

NUTRITION—Vitamins are vital organic compounds that the body is unable to synthesize and which must be supplied by daily food intake. The major diseases of the 19th century, for instance, such as beriberi, pellagra, scurvy and rickets were all directly caused by a lack of specific vitamins and were considered "man-made" in that dietary deficiencies were responsible. The RDA (Recommended Daily Allowance) tables used widely today are merely useful as guidelines and represent much less than the actual amounts of vitamins needed in an adequate diet as they do not allow for a reserve to be built up in the tissues.

Minerals are nonorganic substances necessary to the normal functioning of the body and are not only important by themselves, but also for the way in which they combine with other necessary elements within the body and become an integral part of body structure and function. The ratio of the elements one to the other is a determining factor in good health. There are 28 minerals needed by the human body, of which 14 are present in such small amounts they are termed trace elements.

Honeybee pollen contains all identified vitamins and minerals needed in human nutrition in perfectly balanced amounts and proportions, one to the other.

Remember, if there is a shortage of only one element in the food eaten daily, the body is unable to synthesize or extract what's necessary for proper maintenance and health of the cells and tissue. This applies to all nutrients the body requires, not only vitamin and mineral substances, but also hormones, enzymes, coenzymes, amino acids (protein), carbohydrates and fats. The body is only able to properly use food effectively when there is a complete selection of all necessary elements. The simple addition of honeybee pollen to your diet assures you of the fact that your body is supplied with all nutrients necessary for full, youthful vitality and health. Pollen is a superior source of energy that produces strength in the body, prevents fatigue and builds endurance.

This incredibly complex live natural food is health insurance of a very real kind.

HEALTH—The natural antibiotic in bee pollen has been isolated and found to be extremely active. This may be the reason regular honeybee pollen users are seldom ill. I can't remember the last time I had the flu or even a cold.

Pollen is a giant germ-killer in which bacteria cannot exist; it destroys harmful intestinal flora and provides a strong resistance to infection of any kind.

Bee pollen protects the body against many harmful food additives and environmental poisons found in our food, water and air. It either lessens or completely eliminates the toxic effects of carbon monoxide, ozone and nitrogen dioxide, lead, mercury, DDT, Strontium 90, cadmium, radioactive iodine 131, nitrates and nitrites, some drugs and x-rays.

Dr. Jeffrey S. Bland, Ph.D., and Associate Professor of Chemical and Environmental Science, Tacoma, Washington, notes, "The price we pay for living in the 20th century includes an increase in stress agents." Chemical food additives, toxic environmental substances like asbestos, ozone and other debilitating agents abound in our polluted air. Artificial flavors and colors, stabilizers, preservatives, emulsifiers and other food chemicals are also a form of pollution in a sense. Dr. Bland cautions, "Most of these compounds place an unknown amount of stress on our physiology. When the process of tissue building falls behind that of tissue destruction, then the body will be in a state of biochemical and physiological regression leading potentially to disease."

X-rays, an admittedly valuable diagnostic tool, and radiotherapy treatment for cancer, for example, enter the body with ionizing radiation. Irradiation irreversibly damages cells, as does the natural aging process, but at a highly accelerated pace.

Dr. Peter Hernuss, University of Vienna, Austria, conducted a study of 25 women with inoperable uterine cancer. Some of the women received pollen and it was found that the natural antibodies increased in this group, with a higher concentration of leukocytes and infection-fighting red blood cells also being recorded. The pollen-fed group suffered less from the side effects of the treatments, such as nausea, insomnia, hair loss and inflammation. The control group receiving a placebo did not experience relief.

Any serious study of the benefits of honeybee pollen reveals astounding cures of nearly every condition of ill-health and disease known to man. Unfortunately, much of this research is conducted outside the United States and has not received the widespread notice it deserves.

From France, most notably Dr. Remy Chauvin and Dr. Edouard Lenor Mand, Managing Trustee of the Institute of Bee Culture and the Paris Child Preventatorium respectively, we hear of bee pollen being used successfully in the treatment of chronic constipation or diarrhea, false diarrhea with bloody mucus, colibacillose, diverticulosis, acute crisis of articular rheumatism with cardiac complications and deteriorating lymphatic conditions, intestinal kidney disease, liver complaints, premature aging and senility, inflamed intestines and/or infection of the large intestine, as a restorer of the growth factor after serious illness and in anemia and rickets, with the bee pollen treatments causing a 30% increase in hemoglobin count.

A German/Swedish urology team reported the successful treatment of prostate condition in over 170 cases. Surgical intervention was not needed.

Two gerontologists of the USSR have been testing pollen for a number of years and state pollen causes cell-rejuvenation and aids in the formation of new tissue. They conclude pollen ingestion adds years to the life-span.

In the U.S., Dr. Kilmer McCully of Harvard Medical School discovered that heart disease is often initiated by a deficiency of pyradoxin (Vitamin B6) and an increase of methionine. Foods with a high B6 and low methionine ratio may prevent some forms of heart disease. Bananas have a ratio of 40 to 1, carrots 15 to 1—but honeybee pollen has a ratio of 400 to 1. Honeybee pollen wins again.

In England, Dr. Gordon Latto treats his hay fever patients suffering allergy attacks with pollen-laden honey and reports amazing results.

Dr. Leo Conway, Denver, Colorado, by 1972 had treated thousands of documented and verified cases of allergies with pollen itself successfully. (Hay fever sufferers are affected by the anemophile, or windborn pollens, not the heavier entomophile pollens gathered by the bees.)

The astounding ability of honeybee pollen to balance body chemistry, thus allowing the body to cure itself naturally, appears to be the active "ingredient" in bee pollen's amazingly successful treatment of so many widely diverse conditions of ill health.

ATHLETES—Athletes report, and I can personally verify, that bee pollen increases stamina to a remarkable degree. Steve Riddick, billed as the "fastest man on earth," has been taking pollen since 1974. He says that after just two months he felt, "as if my body shifted into a more powerful gear." This is a wonderful description of the invincible feeling bee pollen imparts to the user. I agree with him 100%. A two-year research program conducted by Remi Korchemny at the Pratt Institute in New York provides a scientific basis for the fact that bee pollen does improve the crucial recovery power of athletes.

BEAUTY—The ladies may be interested to know that Lars-Erik Essen, a Swedish dermatologist, has been researching the beauty benefits of pollen for some time. He reports that pollen prevents premature aging of the skin cells, by stimulating growth of new skin tissue. It protects against dehydration and smooths away wrinkles with the skin becoming smoother and healthier.

French scientists report their research shows pollen can actually reverse the aging of the skin and fade away age spots. Pollen also exercises a suppressive effect on acne.

WEIGHT CONTROL—Pollen, the wonder food, also aids in natural weight control by correcting any chemical imbalance in the metabolism. It causes a fast increase in the rate of calorie burning and contains 15% lecithin, the natural substance that melts away fat. The real wonder of this incredible food is that it can be helpful when weight gain is needed also, simply by correcting the metabolic balance in the body.

IMPOTENCE—By far the most stupendous impact bee pollen made in my life was making possible my return to sexual potency at age 71, an unheard of happening, as far as the medical men are concerned. I credit this directly to the gonadatropic hormone present in live bee pollen. This hormone is similar to the pituitary hormone, gonadotropin, and feeds the sex glands, acting as a stimulant. This is a natural sex hormone and nourishes the reproductive systems of both men and women increasing sexual stamina and endurance, and has been found to have a dramatic effect on sexual ability.

I am not the only person in the world who has been returned to full manhood by the simple ingestion of honeybee pollen. This is not an isolated occurrence. German medical doctors have reported the increase of up to double the hormone count in patients fed one teaspoon of pollen every morning over a period of only three to six weeks. In most cases, the improvement could be measured by three weeks, but in even the most stubborn cases, the hormone count had doubled by six weeks.

Research conducted in Yugoslavia with a group of impotent men fed pollen resulted in over half showing a definite improvement in sperm production and sexual performance in just one month.

A California couple, she now aged 90 and he 84 years of age, are a inspiring example of the power of pollen. As a former nurse, the wife was aware of the importance of good nutrition and the proper feeding of the glands. She and her husband, then 81 and impotent for over fifteen years, began eating bee pollen daily. After a time they were delighted to find they were able to resume full normal sexual activity and are continuing to enjoy intimate relations to this day. They report the same happy result in six other men, all over 80, with whom they shared the good news and who are now taking pollen daily themselves. An interesting side-effect was noted in the original couple. The husband was able to discard the corrective eye-glasses he had used for 44 years. He simply didn't need them anymore.

CONCLUSION—Although I began by eating fresh, raw bee pollen as a supplement to my diet, I now carry High Desert® pollen tablets with me wherever I go. These tablets contain a homeopathic 130 mg of raw High Desert® pollen and have been scientifically formulated to "pollenize" or balance the three pounds of food eaten daily by the average adult.

Research conducted by the USDA in 1946, (as reported in the Journal of the National Cancer Institute, Vol. 9, No. 2, October 1948), showed that pollenized food of one part to 10,000 either prevented or delayed the appearance of mammary tumors. Existing tumors were reduced in size. Later experiments conducted by equally authoritative sources confirmed that this percentage of bee pollen to food is the perfect homeopathic amount.

My tablets contain no chemical additives or sugar, only pure and natural ingredients. Extra-High Potency™ High Desert® Honeybee PollenS™ tablets are both chewable, making them easy to take anytime I need a quick energy lift, and good-tasting as well. They are formed by a completely cold process to retain full nutrient value and do not require refrigeration. They are made for me by the C C Pollen Company of Scottsdale, Arizona, the largest harvester of honeybee pollen in the United States and I recommend them highly.

You can confidently expect a miracle in your life when you start eating honeybee pollen daily.

QUICK QUESTIONS & ANSWERS ON BEE POLLEN

Questions I'm Most Often Asked

Everywhere I go, wherever I speak, on every talk-show, and even in coversation with friends, I am asked about bee pollen. It seems everyone wants to know more about the world's only perfect food, this miracle from the beehive.

Remember, I'm only answering for High-Desert® pollen products. These are the finest, in my opinion, and the only kind I eat. They are live and potent. I can't answer for any others on the market, but, to my way of thinking, the others are not in the natural-food category because of either where they are harvested, or how they are handled and processed.

Although the preceding chapter on pollen treats the subject in depth, here are the questions I'm most often asked, along with my answers—short and snappy.

Q—What is bee pollen? A—Pollen is the male seed of the plant that must be joined with the female element for reproduction. Bees fly from one plant to another gathering the pollen for the hive and fertilizing each flower as they buzz along. Every small speck of pollen has all the ingredients to reproduce life. That means it has all the vitamins, minerals, enzymes, coenzymes, amino acids (protein), carbohydrates, hormones and trace elements and is a powerhouse of energy for the human body.

Q—Is bee pollen the excretion of the bee? A—Of course not. I can't understand why anyone would think that. The bees gather the live pollen from the inside of the flowers.

Q—Where does bee pollen come from? A—The bees gather the pollen from flowers and store it in their hive for future food. A beekeeper places a pollen-trap on the hive and as the bees enter the colony, they must pass through a series of screens. The screens gently brush part of the pollen off and it falls into the pollen drawer. The beekeeper harvests the pollen from the drawer. Since more pollen is collected than the bees need, we don't harm the colony by taking a portion for our use.

Q—Does bee pollen really work? A—It sure does! In ancient times, people throughout the world used pollen-laden raw honey and pollen itself for its energy-giving, life-prolonging medicinal qualities. Medical doctors in foreign countries are using pollen regularly for treatment of many conditions of ill-health with great success. Athletes around the globe have increased their performance by eating pollen. I myself, at age 86, eat bee pollen every day to keep well and continue my strenuous activities. The only food that has every element the body needs can't help but work.

Q—Do you eat bee pollen? A-Well, I should say I do. I eat bee pollen everyday, several times each day. I don't think there is anything in the world I could use to replace it.

Q—So many health authorities don't practice what they preach—do you? A—You bet! If I didn't, I wouldn't be able to do all the things I do now at 86 years of age. If you do what I do, then I say you should be as I am. I don't know of anyone who preaches and teaches health that has proof what they say is the truth, but I think I'm a pretty good example of what my program accomplishes.

Q—Why haven't we heard much about bee pollen

before? A—Bee pollen's benefits are quite well-known abroad and it's used extensively. Maybe the practitioners of modern medicine in the U.S. would rather give us pills and chemicals for our aches and pains than teach us the importance of natural living as was intended by our Creator. But I predict a major breakthrough in self-care health-care as more and more people learn of this perfect food.

Q—What does bee pollen do for you? A—Well, it certainly gives me the stamina and endurance I need for all my physical activities, plus it keeps me well with natural antibiotic and antiputrefactive properties. I feel great—like everyone should feel, but too many don't. I get up in the morning and get going and whatever I want to do, I can do. I no longer sit around wondering what I'm able to do.

Q—How do you eat pollen? A—I eat both the fresh granules and the natural tablets. Seems I like the raw granules best, but I carry my own-formula tablets with me, especially when I'm making a trip somewhere, and munch on those. Both forms take care of the body, but some folks like the taste of the tablets better.

Q—How should I start eating bee pollen? A—If you haven't eaten High-Desert® pollen before, it's the richest and most potent on the market, take just one or two granules, or 1/4 of a tablet, and put it under your tongue. Let it dissolve and you'll find out your body's reaction. Some people can't eat even one strawberry—or take penicillin—without a reaction, it may be the same with some people and pollen. Chances are, you won't have a reaction, but it's best to introduce this live potent substance to your body slowly. Next day, eat a little more and you'll soon know what you should take.

Q—What kind of reaction should I look out for? A—Probably none, but a very small percentage may experience watery, itchy eyes, flushing or a slight nausea and an occasional gas pain. A minute percentage could experience shortness of breath or difficulty breathing. If you have any allergies or serious health problems, see your doctor before taking pollen.

For every one report we get from a person who has difficulty taking pollen, we have a veritable flood of grateful letters from people telling the benefits pollen has brought to them. Pollen helps more people than it harms. Should we outlaw strawberries or penicillin because of the few who have a reaction?

We know there are many low-strength pollens and pollen-products on the market that cause no "reaction" whatsoever in the body when ingested. We have had reports of a public broadcast in California warning the listening audience that Extra-High Potency High-Desert® bee pollen is an extremely strong and potent food. They cautioned listeners not to take "too much" of our full-strength pollen for fear of having a "reaction." We certainly hope so!

It's true that pollen that has been heated, chemically processed and improperly stored is a "dead" food and will cause no "reaction." The live, full potency of bee pollen will indeed cause a "reaction" in the body—an exciting, energizing rejuvenation of every cell. It is precisely because we know the strength of our High-Desert® pollen that every package carries explicit instructions to begin slowly and monitor your body while taking.

A "reaction" is only the outward manifestation of a sensitivity to the chemical changes that pollen makes in your body. Beginning slowly and building up your daily intake is the way to overcome this sensitivity so that you can experience the benefits of pollen. See your local health food store and sample this miraculous food for yourself.

Q–Can I have a bad reaction from pollen? A–As I explained above, very few people have a "bad reaction" from pollen. Since I've been taking bee pollen and studying up on it, I only know of two instances. In both cases, the "reaction" was directly traceable to the fact that the person started out by taking too much too soon. One person ate a half cupful. This is a live and incredibly potent substance, as proven by the fact that it can make chemical changes in the body. It should be treated with respect.

Q–I understand if you're not careful, pollen can kill you. Is this true? A–Well, I don't think pollen can kill you. Good food will not kill anyone. I've never heard of anyone O.D.ing on pollen, but I suppose it's possible.

Q–Should I continue taking vitamins while eating bee pollen? A–No. You don't need vitamins while you're eating bee pollen. Bee pollen has all the vitamins and minerals and other nutrients you need. If you're eating bee pollen and taking vitamins at the same time, there may not be a balance there. You may get too much of one element and not enough of another. To keep a proper balance in your system, you don't need anything but the pollen.

Q–How will I know if I'm taking the right amount? A–I think the "right" amount depends on how physically active you are. Considering that I get out and train for a 26-mile marathon, or do a 10-mile run for exercise, I may need more than the average person because my physical demands are greater. But, research shows that only an ounce and a half of the fresh pollen, plus water, can actually sustain life indefinitely, and one or two 130 mg tablets daily are sufficient to produce positive results. My best answer is that pollen is a food, not a drug. You must listen to your body and judge your own "right" amount personally.

Q—What's the difference between fresh pollen granules and bee pollen tablets? A—Just about the same differences as between a bunch of grapes or a handful of raisins. Bee pollen tablets are just the concentrated form of fresh pollen granules. Some people don't like the taste of pollen so they won't eat it, even though they know it's good for them. Chewable pollen tablets taste good and are an easy, convenient way to add pollen to your daily diet. You can also take bee pollen capsules of straight granules.

Q—When will I start feeling the effects of taking pollen? A—Evidence of pollen ingestion has been found in the blood, urine and even the spinal fluid within one to two hours after eating. I take my bee pollen first thing in the morning and I think I start feeling it immediately. People say the first noticeable effect is an increase in energy and well-being, with less need for sleep. Improvement in digestion is usually noticed within a week or two. Pollen has a cumulative building effect and you need to take it regularly for a period of time to fully experience all benefits.

Q—Can I take too much pollen? A—Pollen is a good food, and while you can't take "too much," you can take more than you need. One of the biggest mistakes many people make is eating more food in general than the body actually requires. If your body is not deficient in any elements and your level of physical activity is average, a tablespoon or two of the fresh granules and/or one or two tablets daily is all that's needed to produce positive results.

Q—Is High-Desert® pollen clean? A—Certainly. It's perfectly clean. The beekeeper screens his pollen harvest into a poly-lined container and immediately freezes it until shipment to the C C Pollen Company cleaning facility. There the pollen is mechanically cleaned using specially designed equipment. It is then packaged and held at zero degrees until shipment to the store or consumer.

Q–Is High-Desert® pollen treated with chemicals? A–Absolutely not! It is a live, fresh product and this freshness is preserved by freezing, not artificial or chemical preservatives. Adding stabilizers and chemical preservatives would increase the keeping qualities for a year or so, but it would no longer be the fresh, live and potent food it is now. Heat-treating kills enzymes and reduces nutrient content, but is used by some companies as a method of preservation. The only satisfactory way to maintain all nutrients live and intact is by freezing.

Q–Are there any reliable sources where you can buy pollen all year long? A–Yes, of course. The C C Pollen Company is the largest harvester, manufacturer and marketer of honeybee pollen products in the United States. Their facilities are more than adequate for maintaining bee pollen shipments year around.

Q–Is bee pollen a cure-all? A–No, but it does stabilize the all-important metabolism and chemical balance of the body, permitting the body to heal itself. A "cure" is nothing but complete health and health is the normal condition of the body. The body rebuilds itself every seven years. If you take pollen for seven years, for instance, I don't see any reason why you won't have a perfect body at the end of that time, providing you follow other rules of good health.

Q–Should I ever take extra bee pollen? A–During times of stress, menstrual periods, for weight loss, unusually heavy physical activity or exertion–yes. When I'm out running long distances, I even carry some pollen tablets with me. If I'm running for two hours or more, I fuel my body with bee pollen while I'm running.

Q—How long will pollen retain its freshness and nutritive value? A—Indefinitely, if frozen or refrigerated. But I say if you keep it in your freezer, it will retain full potency actually for longer than you should have it. If you're eating it every day, purchase only what you will eat up in a few months' time. I keep my fresh pollen in the freezer and take out only what I need for the day.

Q—Are C C Pollen Company products subject to quality control? A—The quality control of their pollen actually starts before it's contracted for by C C Pollen. Bee yards must be in areas free from urban pollution or agricultural spraying. Then each separate pollen-flow is individually tested and evaluated before being accepted for C C Pollen Company products. Pollen tastes and smells different during every pollen-flow, depending on what flowers are in bloom at the time. Also, C C Pollen Company cleaning, packaging and shipping facilities are under inspection by the State Health Department and the FDA also and are the finest and cleanest anywhere.

Q—Then I can rely on C C Pollen Company cleanliness and freedom from impurities and contaminates? A—You betcha! High-Desert® pollens are harvested mostly in the high desert areas where they don't use any fumigation, chemical sprays, insecticides or fertilizers. Everything's natural up there. It can't help but be clean and pure, just the way you want it.

Q—Does fresh bee pollen have to be refrigerated? A—Absolutely. Fresh pollen loses up to 76% of its nutritive value over a year if not refrigerated or frozen. A week or two at room temperature will not cause deterioration though. High-Desert® tablets do not need to be refrigerated and can be conveniently carried in pocket or purse.

Q—What's the best time to eat pollen? A—I take my bee pollen first thing in the morning and a little more whenever I eat. Since pollen has all the nutrients required by the body, this way I know that no matter what I eat with the pollen, I am providing my body with every element it needs to extract, assimilate or synthesize exactly what's required by every cell and gland. If only one element is missing in the food eaten, the body can't make full and effective use of what's provided. I make sure I provide every element needed by eating my pollen.

Q—If I'm allergic to pollen, how can pollen alleviate my allergies? A—Chances are the pollen you're allergic to is the light wind-born pollens, the most common culprit in hay fever. Bees collect the heavier, richer pollens. Taking a little pollen daily will overcome your allergies by providing the same kind of immunization you get from a small pox vaccination, for instance. Many doctors routinely treat allergies by giving minute doses of the allergic substance to successfully build up immunization.

Q—How much does High-Desert® pollen cost? A—High-Desert® pollen tablets are priced at $5 for 30 tablets, and just $10 for 90 tablets—which gives you an extra 30 tablets free. Fresh High-Desert® granules cost about $10 per pound, or $12 per pound if canned for long-term storage. A five-pound package of the fresh granules is just $45 or only $9 per pound.

Q—Why is your High-Desert® pollen so expensive? A—Expensive? Compared to what? High-Desert® pollen isn't expensive. If you went to the health-food store and purchased all the natural (not artificial chemically produced) vitamins, minerals, enzymes, coenzymes, amino acids, carbohydrates, hormones, trace elements and other nutrients in pollen separately, you'd run up quite a bill. Then, when you took so-many units of this and so-many milligrams of that, you probably wouldn't strike the proper balance of elements anyway. Bee pollen has a perfectly proportioned balance of all nutrients.

When you consider what you're getting and what it does for you, it isn't "expensive" at all. It's real "health insurance," too.

Q—How many International Units of the different vitamins are in each ounce of pollen or in one tablet? A—International Units may be useful as a guideline when taking the chemically produced individual vitamins, but they just don't apply to pollen. Too many people today are hung up on taking so-many units of this and so-many units of that, and it just isn't working. What's needed is the balanced and perfectly proportioned nutrients in bee pollen.

Q—Well then, how much of the Recommended Daily Allowance of each vitamin are present in each ounce of pollen or one tablet? A—It's the chemical balance of the body that determines how the vitamins and minerals and other elements in food are used, and whether or not they are used properly and effectively. The RDA tables just can't read each individual chemical make-up and make a generalized evaluation and expect it to be accurate. The only safe method of supplying the body with all the nutrients it requires, that I've discovered anyway, is by eating bee pollen every day.

Q—What makes Extra-High Potency™ High-Desert® pollen extra-high potency? A—The pollens in Extra-High Potency™ High-Desert® PollenS™ are a superior blending of pollens harvested in the high deserts and elsewhere. Continuing research shows that a blend of bee pollens from many areas is superior to any single-source pollen, richer and more potent. Flash-freezing at zero degrees assures full nutrient value is maintained, along with the high potency present at the moment of harvest.

Q—How can I identify quality pollen? A—The fresher, the better. Many pollens are packaged, sealed and allowed to sit on a shelf for an indefinite length of time with chemical preservatives to keep them from spoiling. Anything added to the pollen to keep it from spoiling reduces the quality. The only satisfactory method of preservation is freezing or refrigerating fresh pollen. The tablets should be made with only pure and natural ingredients, nothing chemical or artificial. C C Pollen Company products meet my rigid requirements.

Q—I suffer from diabetes, hypoglycemia, cancer, arthritis, impotence, heart disease. Can I take pollen? A—When people come to me and say they have one of the killing or disabling diseases, my heart goes out to them. I know the helpless feeling they are experiencing. I tell them, yes, I believe you can safely take pollen by taking just a little to start with to test the body's reaction. As far as your condition is concerned, why I believe bee pollen is just what you need. Some prescribed drugs seem to have so many harmful side effects, they do as much damage as they do good, to my way of thinking. They used to say, "it's something you ate" when something went wrong with the body. More likely, it's something you didn't eat. The ability of pollen to correct any imbalance in the body's chemistry and restore normal functioning, allowing the body to heal itself, may be just what you need.

Q—I've been informed that I should only eat pollen from my local area. Is this true? A—No. I believe in a great variety of everything. Besides studies show that a mixture or blend of pollens is superior to pollen from one area anyway. It's much more beneficial to eat a blending of pollens from many states and areas, like High-Desert® .

Q—I find High-Desert® pollen is much more costly than Spanish pollen. Why is that? A—Let me count the ways High-Desert® is better! Let's look at the way Spanish pollen is harvested, handled, processed and shipped. Many foreign pollens are fumigated to retard bacteria growth and almost all are baked to reduce moisture content. Besides that, it's old by the time it gets here. And it's preserved like a box of chemically processed cereal is preserved, so it will keep for a long time. It is much less expensive to dump in a bunch of chemicals, package the stuff, and ship it here to sit on a shelf with no refrigeration, than it is to harvest and maintain the full potency and nutritive value of High-Desert® pollen. You choose. You can eat handfuls of foreign pollen that's been processed in this manner and you'll find no reaction or chemical changes occurring in your body whatsoever.

At 86, I've seen the introduction of paved walks, roads and freeways, electric lights, radios, television, automobiles, planes, jets, missiles, various bombs and so on—all material progress only. This is on the "outside." What progress have we made on the "inside?" Very little. In fact, we have deteriorated as a race in many ways. I see progress being made now on the "inside"—with bee pollen becoming more and more available and its benefits recognized.

The World-Famous

DR. RINSE FORMULA

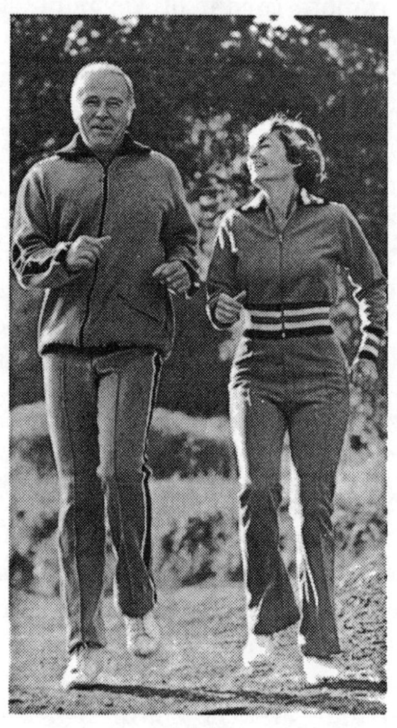

This amazing formula, developed by Dr. Rinse for his personal use after an incapacitating heart attack, has overcome heart disease in tens of thousands of individuals around the world. Empirical evidence in the form of testimonials from grateful users shows the Dr. Rinse Formula not only aids in the fight against cardiovascular and circulatory problems by cleaning out arteries clogged with cholesterol, but can reduce high blood pressure and even eases the pain of arthritis.

JACOBUS RINSE, Ph.D.
THE MAN HIMSELF

Luke 4:23 "Physician, heal thyself"

I became personally acquainted with Jacobus Rinse one crisp Sunday afternoon in the middle of his vast acreage in a remote corner of Vermont. My wife and I motored up from our home to have dinner at his invitation. We drove leisurely, thoroughly enjoying our passage through the rolling hills of Ohio, ablaze with the changing colors of autumn, up through the majestic mountains of Pennsylvania crowned with snow-caps and wreathed with hazy clouds of snow.

Following the good doctor's excellent directions, we finally reached the Rinse holdings and turned into the lane. As we drove down what has to be the longest "driveway" I ever traveled, we heard the sound of a chain-saw echoing across the river. As we continued driving down the lane, the sound got louder and we were busy looking around trying to spot the operator through the trees when the saw noise stopped.

Suddenly, coming across the river toward the road, there appeared Dr. Jacobus Rinse. I stopped the car and walked eagerly to greet him. I found it hard to believe this alert, vigorous man coming toward me with the welcoming smile was 84 years old. His stride was that of a much younger man and the chain-saw in his hand testified to his afternoon's occupation. "Just clearing out some dead wood," he explained. "I was cutting it into lengths to fit the fireplace and stacking it into cords."

After a very pleasant and convivial meal, I expressed my surprise and complimented him on his excellent physical condition. Even though I had read his published works and many of the articles written about him, I still was amazed to think he had transformed himself from a semi-invalid who, according to his medical prognosis, should have been dead long ago, into the dynamo seated before me.

He chuckled a little and told us a bit about his schedule. On many occasions, he said, he climbs into his old Volkswagen and makes the four-hour trip down to New York City in his capacity as chemical consultant. Upon arriving in the city, he may give a lecture, attend a luncheon or participate in a meeting. Without staying overnight or pausing to rest, he then climbs into the VW and makes the four-hour return trip. Dr. Rinse regularly works until 2:00 in the morning and boasts, in his words, "a heart as sound as a child's."

Although many people are unaware of it, the Dr. Rinse Formula he developed, and which has helped so many overcome their health problems, brings him no income. This remarkable man has no commercial interest in the preparation and accepts no remuneration whatsoever. It is strictly an altruistic effort. Dr. Jacobus Rinse is a benefactor of mankind and, as a healer, knows no peer.

When asked if he had any secrets, he smiled in reply. "No secrets. Proper nutrition, suitable exercise and my formula, that's all." Dr. Rinse says emphatically, "Anyone can have the same results."

IN THE BEGINNING

Thirty-four years ago, after suffering his first heart attack at the age of 51, Dr. Jacobus Rinse was told he had ten years to live—provided he restricted all physical activity and took his prescribed medications daily. Remembering the sharp pain and agonizing vice-like constriction of the chest he experienced during his heart seizure, which followed an unusually active weekend clearing the land where his new house was to stand, Dr. Rinse resolved to follow the orders of his cardiologist to the letter. With his very life at stake, he had too much to lose to take any chances whatsoever. His life as a virtual invalid began.

Born and educated in Holland and holding a doctorate in physical chemistry, Dr. Rinse couldn't understand what factors had combined to create his heart condition. As a textbook case, he didn't fit. By medical standards, he should not have been a candidate for early heart problems. He knew that individuals at risk usually have a family history of heart disease, that many smoke, and that most are over-weight and eat a diet high in cholesterol. Dr. Rinse was the first member of his family to experience a heart attack, had never smoked and watched his diet, virtually eliminating foods targeted as high in cholesterol, such as eggs, butter, most dairy products and fatty meats. Other contributing factors to heart disease are thought to include physical strain to the breaking point and emotional stress or excitement continuing over a period of time. He examined his life and found these criteria did not apply to him either.

Yet, in spite of his healthy lifestyle, his angina attack was the very real result of an atherosclerotic condition characterized by cholesterol-clogged arteries. Popping nitroglycerin pellets, sometimes as often as every fifteen or thirty minutes, to open up the constricted arteries which caused his heart to spasm painfully, was not to his liking. Dr. Rinse explains, "I was not satisfied to make use of these small pellets for the rest of my life—even if it was only to be 10 years."

As a practicing research chemist, Dr. Rinse determined to change his body chemistry and reverse his prognosis. He started investigating natural foods thought to protect against cholesterol buildup and began eating raw foods rich in fat-liquifying enzymes. From 1951 when he suffered his first heart failure until 1957, he lived on raw fruits, raw vegetables, raw herring, raw meat, raw eggs and yogurt. He began taking 1000 mg of Vitamin C (ascorbic acid) daily and a multivitamin tablet. Being aware of the research of Evan Shute, M.D. and Wilfrid E. Shute, M.D. of Ontario, Canada who successfully treated many heart patients with Vitamin E, he determined to follow their recommendations and began taking 200 mg of Vitamin E after meals.

During this period, Dr. Rinse relates that the one single supplement he felt helped him best tolerate increased physical activity was *garlic*. (Editor's Note: See Section II.) Talking of the rigid regimen he set for himself and followed without deviation for six long years, Dr. Rinse now says, "By avoiding overly strenuous exercise, I managed to live a more or less normal life."

However, his satisfactions were few and in 1957, he experienced another excruciating attack, lasting an agonizing hour this time.

He suffered almost constant spasms of angina pain, in spite of his medication. His heart-rate rose an alarming 50 beats and he was slow to recover after the slightest amount of exercise. It was beginning to appear the medical experts were right after all.

With six years of his precious projected ten gone, Dr. Rinse refused to be conquered and began his serious research all over again. There had to be a key.

Certain scientific tests conducted on laboratory animals with chemically-induced high cholesterol levels came to his attention. This research indicated the substance *lecithin,* derived from soybeans, could actually dissolve cholesterol. In addition, *safflower oil* was shown to contain precisely the polyunsaturated fatty acids needed to reduce cholesterol to a liquid state. Could it be possible that a combination of lecithin and safflower oil would conquer atherosclerosis in humans and clear clogged arteries? Dr. Rinse decided to find out, using himself as a guinea pig.

Along with his other supplements, he began to take one tablespoon each of lecithin and safflower oil daily. Incredible as it may sound, in only a *few days,* he began to feel the difference as his body responded.

Dr. Rinse reported, "My angina pains ceased. My galloping pulse rate decreased slightly, but noticeably. Excellent results began to appear within a few days." After three months of continued use, his angina symptoms totally disappeared, even after exercise. The chemist in him attributed his improvement to the lecithin and safflower oil.

One short year later, his physical activity now encompassing even heavy outside work, his condition appeared completely cured. Dr. Rinse explained, "I am convinced the food supplement I developed is both a preventive and cure for atherosclerosis. I have had no recurrence of angina or other diseases. It seems the atherosclerotic plaques which had been narrowing my arteries to cause heart failure have been reversed."

Judging from his extraordinary health at 84 years of age, Dr. Jacobus Rinse was completely correct. He has personally conquered one of the major killers of our time.

THE DR. RINSE FORMULA A PERSONAL ACCOUNT

Recently, my mother-in-law, 69, frail, with a weak heart, suffering from atherosclerosis and angina pain, crippled and all but incapacitated by arthritis and osteoporosis, took it into her sweet stubborn head to leave her native Bavaria and come to the United States to visit us. My wife was frantic with worry over her condition and certain the trip would end with our having to put her in a hospital. She prayed only that it wouldn't happen en route, with Nan-Nan being rushed on an emergency basis to a hospital in some distant city.

We tried every which way to change Nan-Nan's mind, including several *very* long-distance phone calls, but it didn't matter to her that we had a trip scheduled to see her the coming autumn and offered to escort her back with us; it didn't matter to her that her health really wasn't up to such a long trip and she refused to confront the possibility of a fall which could result in broken bones already weakened by her osteoporosis.

Osteoporosis is a very common condition in the elderly, especially those living alone. It is caused by a disturbance of the body's metabolism resulting from a deficiency of certain nutrients and minerals (primarily calcium), usually present in an adequate diet. But, like many senior citizens, Nan-Nan's family had scattered. With no one to cook for but herself, we were sure she had lost interest in food and no longer bothered to serve herself a balanced meal. Without the elements they need to keep strong, bone mass and density decrease, the bone becomes honeycombed with too much air space and osteoporosis progresses rapidly. Such bones are brittle, fragile and break very easily.

Nan-Nan had already undergone two separate operations for joint replacement when her brittle bones had snapped and would not heal. She was in constant pain from angina and the osteoporosis, and favored her right side when she walked, creating a back problem as well.

Nan-Nan's angina attacks required strong medication to bring the pain to bearable levels. The coronary insufficiency she labored under was caused by an advanced case of atherosclerosis, commonly called "hardening of the arteries," often making her short of breath as her heart labored to send oxygenated blood where it was needed. With the blood flow to her heart slowed by constricted and ever-narrowing blood vessels, she was a prime candidate for a heart attack, stroke or other degenerative condition—all of which come from atherosclerosis.

Add to that the swollen joints and nodules of the arthritis that cruelly curled her hands and sent pains shooting through her body and you can well understand why we were worried about Nan-Nan making such a long trip alone.

Always indomitable, Nan-Nan let us know she was determined to come alone *now*—and that's exactly what she did. The relief was evident on my wife's face when we met the plane and she could finally put her arms around the tiny hobbling figure and support her to the car. Her face was gray with the fatigue of the long flight, but we got her home and I tucked her up warm and cozy while my wife went to fetch a cup of herb tea and honey for all of us.

Leaving them to chat a little, I took my tea downstairs to my favorite chair and began to think seriously about Nan-Nan's medical problems. Certainly it was going to be easy to make sure she had an adequate diet while she was with us, but she refused to leave her home-place and live with any of her children. What would happen to her health when she went back home? What single one thing could we do for her that was simple and easy enough for her to continue when she returned to Bavaria? What could we do in the four short months of her visit that would make enough difference in the way she felt so that she would *want* to continue it herself? Suddenly it came to me! Nan-Nan would join us in taking the *Dr. Rinse Formula breakfast-mash* every day.

Two years before when I was entering my 50s, I found I was slowing down and I didn't like it. I had always followed what are generally considered good health practices and enjoyed robust good health for the whole of my life, but I suddenly found myself puffing going up the stairs and continually fell asleep after dinner. Although there wasn't anything I could really put my finger on, except shortness-of-breath and lack of energy, I took myself to the doctor. He joked I was "just getting old," but put me through a complete battery of tests. He found my cholesterol levels were elevated above the normal range and talked to me about "hardening of the arteries" and what medical problems atherosclerosis could create.

In 1983, I had presented "The Dr. Rinse Formula" to my readers. I was personally very impressed with the good doctor and his natural nutritional almost-miraculous cures of atherosclerosis, high (and low) blood pressure, arthritis, bursitis, phlebitis, angina and more. I recalled such a flood of letters from grateful individuals testifying joyously to their renewed well-being and health after taking Dr. Rinse's Formula, it created a happy problem—that of selecting just a few to excerpt for publication! The very thing for me, I thought to myself.

From that time on, my wife and I began taking Dr. Rinse's breakfast-mash religiously. My cholesterol reading fell dramatically and I have the boundless energy of a child again. My wife glows and the twinges of early arthritis she was experiencing have vanished. Apparently we had caught ourselves in time, but what about Nan-Nan? Could Dr. Rinse's Formula help such a diversity of medical problems all concentrated in one frail old body?

YES! The very next morning, with a little urging from my wife, Nan-Nan downed her portion of Dr. Rinse's Formula and dutifully took the alfalfa tablets I laid out for her. Although her problems were of very long-standing, I am absolutely delighted to report that within just two weeks, changes in her condition were noticeable. Her breathing was no longer labored and she seemed to be getting around more comfortably. Within two short months, she was able to help around the house—and enjoyed it thoroughly. By the time she left to return home after four months with us, she was freely moving her fingers without pain for the first time in eight years, thanks to the Rinse Formula and the alfalfa tablets!

It is impossible to fully describe the dramatic changes Dr. Rinse's Formula worked for Nan-Nan. We brought home a fragile, stooped old lady suffering from a seemingly impossible conglomeration of ills and sent home a relatively spry happy oldster looking forward to life again! Her last letter says she is doing marvelously and confirms she will never be without her breakfast-mash. I, for one, am not surprised! Chalk up another victory for Dr. Rinse.

NUTRITION FOR A HEALTHY HEART

Why the Rinse Formula Works

According to the most recent Vital Statistics report as tabulated and compiled by the United States government, nearly three-quarters of American deaths can be traced to four causes: cancer, stroke, accidents and *heart disease*. The National Center for Health Statistics report for the year 1982 shows that 326 persons died of heart disease out of every 100,000 Americans that year, making heart disease the major killer of our civilization. Orthodox medical treatment, notably the attempt to regulate serum cholesterol levels, does not appear able to stem the tide.

IS CHOLESTEROL THE CULPRIT?—Cholesterol is an organic compcund of the steroid family and occurs either free or as esters of fatty acids in practically all animal tissues. *Cholesterol is the raw material from which the body produces bile acids, steroid hormones and provitamin D3.* Cholesterol makes up about 3/10th of one percent of weight in the average person. It isn't the cholesterol in the blood that creates the problem, it's whether or not the body has the other materials needed to process it properly.

ATHEROSCLEROSIS—WHAT IS IT?—The old-fashioned term *hardening of the arteries* says it all. If atherosclerotic plaques injure the artery lining, cholesterol and other fats build up on the arterial walls narrowing the passageway and impeding the flow of oxygenated blood. When this happens, the individual is at risk and will most likely suffer a heart attack, stroke or phlebitis. Because it has been clinically determined that an excessive amount of cholesterol in the blood can cause atherosclerosis, medical science has targeted cholesterol as a major factor in heart disease.

CAN CHOLESTEROL BE CONTROLLED BY

DIET?—Science has shown that the amount of cholesterol consumed in the daily diet does not determine the amount of serum cholesterol levels in the blood. The body itself can manufacture up to about 1.5 grams of cholesterol per day. *If cholesterol in the diet is reduced, the body simply increases its manufacture.* Research has shown that diets low in cholesterol are often ineffective in reducing serum cholesterol levels.

What about cholesterol-lowering drugs? A study conducted with 8,000 heart patients on the so-called cholesterol-lowering drugs over a seven year period of time did not result in a lowering of the projected death-rate. The cost of this experimental investigation was over forty million dollars and none of the drugs showed a favorable influence on the death rate.

Many authorities are now taking a second look at the theory which forbids heart patients or those considered at-risk of heart disease the dietary delights of such highly nutritious and common foods as butter, milk, eggs, beef and so on. The basis for this theory is the fact that these foods contain cholesterol-producing saturated animal fats. However, they all *also* contain more than enough *high-density lipoproteins* (HDL) to keep cholesterol in a liquid state.

WHAT ARE "LIPO-PROTEINS?"—Lipoproteins are fat-protein molecules which either carry cholesterol to the tissues, or remove cholesterol from the tissues. It is the *low-density lipoproteins* (LDL) which carry cholesterol *to* the tissues and the *high-density lipoproteins* (HDL) which dissolve and carry cholesterol *away* from the tissues. It has been determined that an important indicator of the possibility of a heart attack is actually the ratio of HDL to LDL. It is therefore desirable to have a high HDL and low LDL ratio.

LECITHIN & LINOLEIC—THE FRIENDLY FATS—Cholesterol can be dissolved in the blood only in the presence of linoleate-lecithin. Because the melting point of cholesterol is 300 degrees F., it is deposited on arterial walls as a insoluble substance at the normal body temperature of 98.6 degrees. However, with the saturated fatty acids of lecithin present, the melting point of cholesterol is reduced to 180 degrees F., still insoluble at body temperature. When linoleate oil is added, the melting point of cholesterol is brought down to 32° F., well below normal body temperature. In a liquid state, cholesterol is not deposited on arterial walls.

A study examining 900 men for atherosclerosis conclusively showed that all *individuals with more than 36% lecithin in their blood had no atherosclerosis.* Individuals with 34% or less lecithin showed evidence of the disease. Because HDL dissolves cholesterol, there is a resulting absence of atherosclerotic plaque, and existing deposits are carried away as well.

THE RINSE FORMULA contains both lecithin and raw sunflower seeds, which provide the necessary linoleate oil.

BREWER'S YEAST & WHEAT GERM—Both Brewer's yeast and wheat germ are particularly good sources of the B vitamins, including inositol and choline. If the body is deficient in these important vitamins, lecithin cannot be produced in adequate amounts. Even a mild deficiency of choline has been shown to decrease the amount of lecithin in the blood and causes less of the cholesterol passing through the liver to be converted into bile. A lack of choline slows down the use of cholesterol in the tissues and encourages heavy fatty deposits in the arteries.

A study conducted with patients recovering from heart attacks confirmed that when choline and inositol were supplemented in the diet, the size of the cholesterol particles and amount of fat in the blood decreased quickly. Within two months, serum cholesterol levels were normal. It must be pointed out that cholesterol cannot be reduced by choline and/or inositol alone, but must be accompanied by lecithin. In addition, lecithin cannot be synthesized in the body without enzymes containing Vitamin B6. These important enzymes, in turn, are active only if magnesium is present.

THE RINSE FORMULA contains debittered Brewer's yeast and wheat germ, both excellent natural sources of choline, inositol and B6.

VITAMIN B6 (PYRIDOXINE)—A low Vitamin B6 level is often characterized by moodiness (or depression if B6 deficiency is severe), nervousness, a feeling of weakness, a lack of energy, water retention and even the inability to remember dreams. Deficiency of B6 often occurs in individuals with a family history of diabetes, celiac disease and hypoglycemia. Some prescription drugs, gastrointestinal disease and radiation therapy deplete the body's stores of B6.

Vitamin B6 is required by the body as a co-enzyme and in metabolic function. It plays a part in protecting the sheath around our nerves and must be present for the body to make efficient use of proteins and amino acids. As does Vitamin C, Vitamin B6 assists in converting amino acids to neurotransmitters (the means brain cells use to communicate with each other). It has been reported to relieve the nausea caused by radiation sickness and the typical morning-sickness of pregnancy. Vitamin B6 has been successfully used in the clinical treatment of arthritis and is reported to reduce the pain and swelling of joints thickened by this disease.

A deficiency of Vitamin B6 has been shown to lead to the development of atherosclerotic plaque. Researchers working under the auspices of MIT found a deficiency of this vital vitamin, especially in conjunction with a high protein diet, can actually cause atherosclerosis. The body converts methionine (an antioxidant amino acid) into homocysteine (an oxidant) which requires B6 to produce cystothionine (a helpful antioxidant). If your diet contains a lot of cooked meat, which produces an excess of methionine, and is also lacking in B6, chances are you are inviting cardiovascular disease.

On the bright side, supplementing the diet with B6 not only assures you are supplying an important nutrient to your heart, but researchers believe B6 can increase energy levels, improve your resistance to stress and may even protect your normal emotional health.

THE RINSE FORMULA contains Vitamin B6 in pure form, plus additional B6 from the wheat germ and yeast. Note: This may be the reason so many arthritics on the Rinse Formula report improvement in their condition as well.

MAGNESIUM—The need for magnesium supplements is magnified by a prolonged siege of diarrhea, a liquid postoperative (or weight-loss) diet, the use of diuretics and the consumption of large amounts of alcohol. A magnesium deficiency often shows itself in irritability, nervousness, foot and leg cramps, muscular weakness—and an irregular heart beat.

An important point to note is that even when Vitamin B6 is present in adequate amounts, a deficiency of magnesium prevents lecithin from forming and slows down the body's use of fats and cholesterol. Research indicates that heart patients given magnesium as a supplement made dramatic improvement and serum cholesterol levels were drastically reduced in just one month.

When serum cholesterol levels are high, the need for magnesium is critical. In a laboratory experiment, rats fed hydrogenated fat and raw cholesterol required sixteen times more magnesium than rats fed a normal diet. When their diet was supplemented with adequate magnesium, however, the rats did not develop atherosclerosis. Even after the arteries were heavily clogged with fatty deposits, adequate magnesium caused cholesterol levels to drop to normal range and the arteries cleared and became healthy.

Further, adequate magnesium levels are shown to fight

stress, help maintain normal muscle contraction ability and aid in the body's adaption to cold. Note: In areas of the country where "soft" water lacking in many minerals exists, science has documented higher magnesium deficiencies.

THE RINSE FORMULA contains the appropriate amount of magnesium needed for heart health.

BONEMEAL (DICALCIUM PHOSPHATE)—Although many foods in the normal diet contain phosphorus, and a lack of phosphorus is rare, calcium is supplied only by various forms of milk. Contrary to popular opinion, even cheeses (unless made with sweet milk) contain little calcium. Authorities believe 2 grams of calcium should be taken daily by the average adult. Unfortunately, because a quart of milk (whole, buttermilk, yogurt, acidophilus) supplies only 1 gram, supplementation is highly desirable for optimum functioning.

A calcium deficiency creates a susceptibility to bone fractures, promotes lower-back pain, a softening of the bones and sets the stage for periodontal disease. If you are on a bed-rest program, are in an orthopedic cast and can't (or don't) exercise, chances are you need additional calcium in your diet. A high-flouride intake, high-protein diets, emotional stress and hard work in high temperatures increase the body's need for calcium. It has long been recognized that nursing mothers and pregnant or menopausal women require extra calcium in their diet.

THE RINSE FORMULA contains the necessary amount of dicalcium phosphate in bonemeal form.

VITAMIN C (ASCORBIC ACID)—Never underestimate the importance of Vitamin C. Those who bruise easily, have excessive dental problems (including spongy bleeding gums), or who suffer tiny hemorrhages of the blood vessels under the skin, commonly known as "spider" veins, may be exhibiting a need for Vitamin C supplementation. An increased need has also been demonstrated in smokers, diabetics, the elderly, allergy victims and individuals under stress.

All animals, including man, must have Vitamin C to survive. Many animals produce Vitamin C in their liver or adrenals, but man lacks the enzyme required in the manufacturing process and must replenish his supply either by a good diet of fresh foods or by supplementation. Vitamin C is needed to guard the brain and spinal cord from free radicals, for connective tissue (collagen) synthesis, for efficient metabolism of fats and carbohydrates, to produce neurotransmitters and for the maintenance of our all-important immune system.

Vitamin C acts as a natural antibiotic, promotes healing, helps maintain healthy gums, keeps the body cooler during exercise, increases energy levels and fights the effects of stress. Many researchers believe Vitamin C offers protection against the common cold and may yet prove to be the answer to the flu.

Vitamin C is also an important ingredient in the management of cholesterol. Research has determined that when HDL and cholesterol reach the liver together, HDL is removed and decomposes. In the presence of Vitamin C, the cholesterol is then converted into bile acids and never reaches the arteries. It passes into the duodenum (portion of the small intestine) where it aids in the emulsification and absorption of fats. As an aid to reduction of serum cholesterol, Vitamin C taken by mouth has been shown to reduce levels of cholesterol in the blood by 35 to 40%.

THE RINSE FORMULA contains the right amount of Vitamin C needed daily by man, both as an aid to cholesterol management and for life.

VITAMIN E (D-ALPHA TOCOPHEROL)—If you suffer from hot flashes, skin problems, muscle cramping, and hands and feet which are always cold (signaling a circulatory problem resulting in insufficient blood flow to the extremities), your body may be trying to tell you something. These are all common symptoms of Vitamin E deficiency.

In addition, Vitamin E is the body's most important fat soluble antioxidant. It protects lipids (fats) in our body from uncontrolled oxidation and free radicals. Oxidation can cause cancer, induce blood clots resulting in heart attack or stroke, and can damage the element in our cells which controls growth, development and aging. Megadosage levels of Vitamin E have been shown to increase resistance to cancer, bacterial and viral infections, stroke, arthritis, heart attack and environmental pollution.

Vitamin E provides substantial protection against heart attacks by preventing abnormal clot formation. Research has shown Vitamin E slows the formation time for abnormal clotting and even prolongs the clotting time of recalcified human plasma. This effect can reduce the incidence of coronary thrombosis in which a clot breaks loose and travels to the heart, resulting in a heart attack. In the literature of the world's medical community, there are over 130 papers supporting the use of Vitamin E in treating and overcoming heart disease.

Vitamin E not only acts as an antioxidant, but promotes a healthy circulatory system, fights environmental toxins and boosts the immune system. Note: Science has determined those who live or work in areas where chemical or environmental pollutants are present in high concentrations have an increased need for Vitamin E.

THE RINSE FORMULA contains Vitamin E in its pure form and also as an element present in wheat germ.

ZINC—A serious zinc deficiency often results in a loss (or diminishing) of the taste sense, usually accompanied by a loss of appetite and the sense of smell. A lack of zinc has also been linked to prostate problems in men over 40 and may contribute to infertility and even diabetes. Low levels of zinc have been shown to slow wound healing and result in a poor resistance to infections as well.

For heart health, zinc is an important mineral which functions as an antioxidant to protect the cell membranes against free radical damage. Science has determined free radical activity increases when inadequate oxygen is supplied to the tissues. Many heart attacks and most strokes can be attributed to poor oxygenation of the blood. Free radical damage often occurs in atherosclerosis because of insufficient circulation. Zinc is one of the specific nutrients which protects the immune system.

THE RINSE FORMULA contains the appropriate amount of zinc, an important antioxidant.

Dr. Rinse's files are bulging with letters and case histories of people from all over the world who have used his nutrient formula to cure cardiovascular disease. Dr. Rinse says, "I developed this formula during seven years of trial and error. Now, because of the overwhelming biochemical evidence in its support and the success with its use, which many hundreds of people in the United States and Europe have reported, I believe strongly in this food supplement formulation I've evolved."

DR. RINSE'S FORMULA PRAISED BY MANY

Here's a Small Sampling from our Files

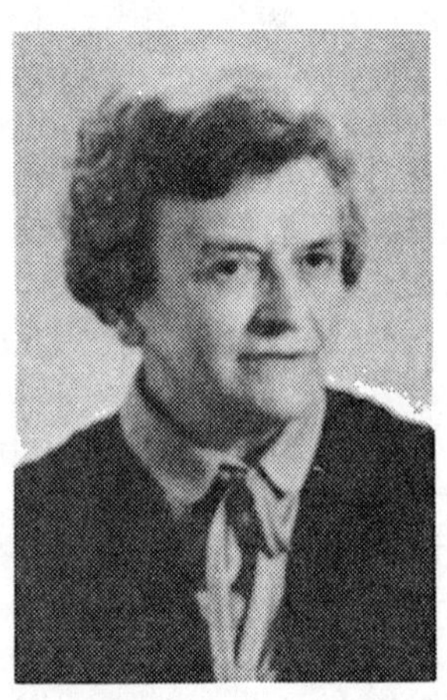

Mrs. Elizabeth Bouse
Housewife
Trenton, New Jersey

Mrs. Bouse, 70 years old, tells us she had been afflicted with swelling of her hands and knuckles and was unable to do any housework for many years. Atherosclerosis and arthritis affected both her knees so severely she was barely able to move around. Even daily chores were beyond her. When a friend told her about it, Mrs. Bouse started taking the Dr. Rinse Formula and three alfalfa tablets three times daily. Her condition began to improve in just two weeks. After two more weeks, her fingers became more flexible and she lost the stiffness in her knees. She was very happy to be able to move around more freely and now rejoices in being able to do her own housework again! After three months on the Dr. Rinse diet, all her symptoms disappeared and she was able to do her daily chores without pain for the first time in many, many years. Mrs. Bouse's doctor was amazed at her improvement and he's now recommending this diet to his patients with similar conditions!

Mrs. Trudy Wein
Billings, Montan

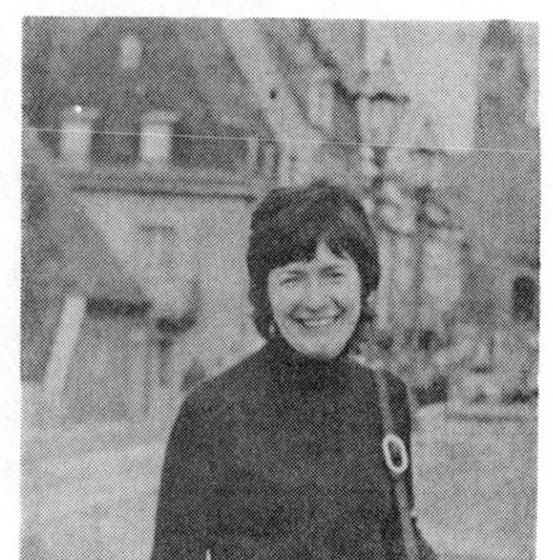

When I turned 40, my doctor put me on medication for various disorders, such as atherosclerosis, arthritis and hypoglycemia (low blood sugar). My blood pressure was always very low and I suffered from cold hands and feet for many years. My fingers and toes felt numb most of the time, except when the arthritic pain caused my fingers to swell and hurt. I took a strong medication which helped my condition somewhat, but at the same time, I became very dizzy, couldn't sleep, had migraine headaches and a sinus condition. A friend of mine read your book and told me about the incredible results she had experienced just by taking the Dr. Rinse breakfast mash. She convinced me. After only a month, I could see the first signs of improvement myself. I'm 45 now and have been using the Dr. Rinse formula for six months. All my symptoms have completely vanished! I can't believe the difference. I can run up the stairs without puffing, my hands and feet are always warm, and my doctor discontinued my medication. Even my cholesterol level is normal. I'm very thankful for this improvement. My doctor now gives me a clean and perfect bill of health. I'm full of energy and everyone thinks I look about ten years younger!

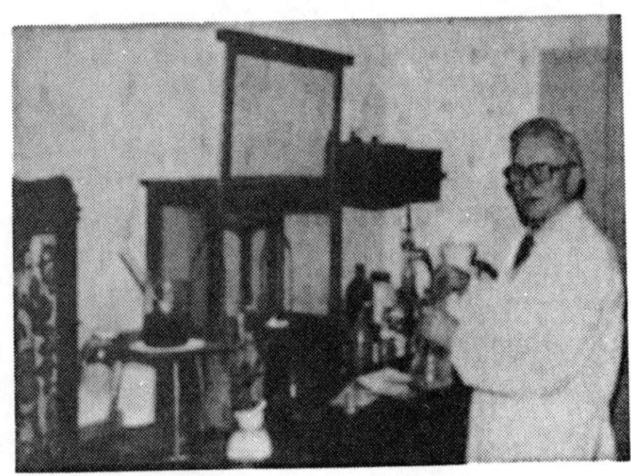

Professor Dr. Armin Hoelscher Chemist and Pharmacist, Retired St. Petersburg, Florida

This 84-year old professional man had severe angina, heart problems, poor blood circulation, very low blood pressure and a high cholesterol level, plus other serious cardiovascular-related ailments. Dr. Hoelscher was unable to walk more than a few hundred yards without stopping frequently to catch his breath. He suffered an artery blockage in his lower right extremities, causing him severe pain. He was forced to drag his right leg as he walked. He was on Lanicor for many years to stabilize his failing heart. After using the Dr. Rinse Formula for just four weeks, he wrote us to say he could feel his symptoms slowly diminishing. After three months on the Dr. Rinse mash, the Professor was able to breathe more freely, could walk up steps without problems and even resumed his morning walks for the first time in many years. After two more months on the mash, Dr. Hoelscher wrote again to tell us of his joy at being able to walk up to two miles daily and do some vigorous exercise and heavy outdoor work. We were especially pleased to hear from this scientist. As a pharmacist and chemist, he was skeptical at first, but is now convinced. What all his other medications were unable to do, the all-natural Dr. Rinse Formula accomplished by providing him all the essentials he needed to stabilize his health!

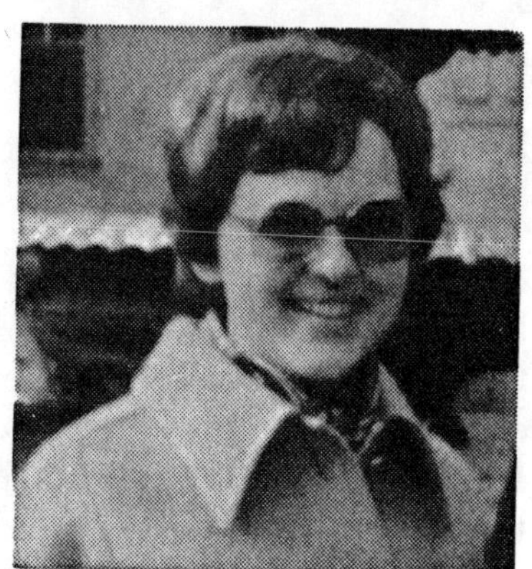

Crystal Fannes
Executive Secretary
Palm Beach, California

At my age of 47, I had always been basically in very good health. But, without any warning, I developed a severe pain in my back caused by blockage of one of my arteries. I also had a very high cholesterol level. While riding in the car with my husband, I suddenly fainted and he rushed me to the hospital. They diagnosed me as having lack of oxygen to the brain, caused by poor circulation. Even my breathing was irregular. My doctor warned me I was a prime candidate for a heart attack if I didn't change my diet. But the medication he gave me seemed to make me feel even worse. I was always tired and had no energy. The world around me was gloomy. After I read about the Dr. Rinse Formula, I mixed it up myself at home and it took only two weeks for me to show improvement. After I had taken the Formula for about four months, I was able to drive again without fear. My family is certainly glad I regained my old happy disposition. I'm not taking my prescribed medication anymore. I don't need it since I've been using Dr. Rinse's mash every day at breakfast. I can't find words strong enough to tell you how thankful I am for your book. I'm full of energy now. My doctor was very surprised to see how fast I recovered my excellent health on the Dr. Rinse Formula.

A.M.H.
Chemist
Borger, Texas

I am 70 years old and hold the equivalent to a major in biology from the University of Missouri. I was the Chief Chemist for Phillip Petroleum during my professional career and am now retired. After reading about Dr. Rinse, I started taking his formula in 1973 with about 2 teaspoons of soy lecithin granules and 1 1/2 teaspoons of safflower oil each morning for breakfast. The mixture was supposed to keep cholesterol in solution so it would not form a slime in the blood vessel which could break loose and plug an artery. At this writing, I have cut back to a rounded teaspoon of lecithin and 1 teaspoon of oil.

After about two years on the Formula, my doctor asked me what I was doing. He said blood tests were like an 18-year old's! After my regular physical exam two years later, he again expressed amazement at my blood tests. after two more years on the breakfast-mash, I took a physical in Temple, Texas and they said the same!

This Formula is so good, it should be publicized to help humanity!

Elna Groth, N.D.
Naturopathic Physician
Austria

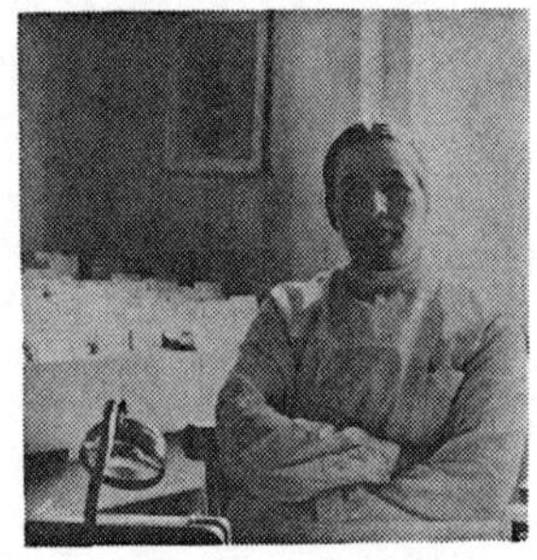

This naturally-oriented health-care professional writes: I'm using strictly homeopathic medicine to take care of my patients' health problems. But sometimes homeopathy doesn't give lasting results and I'm always searching for better treatment for my patients' ailments. While on vacation a few years ago in the U.S., I learned of the Dr. Rinse Formula and have since used it on many hundreds of my patients suffering health conditions that don't normally respond well to any medication. I have seen the most wonderful results with this mixture of vitamins in such cases as heart disease, angina and other coronary problems. Many of my patients afflicted with arthritis, gout, varicose veins, high cholesterol and even eye disorders, such as glaucoma, have responded favorably. I myself have been using Dr. Rinse's mash for almost two years. I must say I feel more energetic and positively rejuvenated! My blood pressure, always a problem is now normalized.

Based on the incredible results I have seen in my patients and the studies on nutrition I have been doing, I feel this formula can overcome the hardships of disease and save many lives. The Dr. Rinse Formula may well be considered a universal health formula for many ailments. I can highly praise it from my own experience. Every person of middle-age should consider the Dr. Rinse mash daily. I believe it may ward off a lot of ailments that might otherwise occur. Dr. Rinse has developed a good, wholesome, natural preventive medicine of the finest kind.

THE DR. RINSE FORMULA

The Proportions Given Below Will Make a
14-Day Supply

7 Tablespoons Lecithin granules
6 Tablespoons raw Wheat Germ
6 Tablespoons debittered Brewer's Yeast (powder or flakes)
6 Tablespoons Sunflower Seeds
6 teaspoons Bonemeal from a reliable source (powder or tablets)
6 Vitamin C tablets of 0.5 grams each
6 Vitamin E tablets (200 International Units total)

TO THESE INGREDIENTS, I ALSO ADD:

6 Tablespoons Bran Flakes (for better bowel movement)
6 teaspoons Kelp powder (or 6-12 Kelp tablets)
12 Zinc Oxide tablets of 10 mg each

All seeds or tablets should first be crushed in a blender.

Blend these ingredients well in a big bowl, stirring until the mixture is uniform. For improved health, take 1 to 2 Tablespoons of the Formula on a daily basis. To insure freshness and complete potency of all ingredients, I recommend you store your Dr. Rinse Formula in a closely covered jar in the refrigerator.

For my personal use, I also add a good dollop (about 1 Tablespoon) of raw, unheated unfiltered honey straight from a friendly neighbor's beehive. You may use molasses, if you prefer. The honey or molasses should be added at the time you swallow the mixture. My morning regimen also includes a good multi-vitamin/mineral tablet and three to five natural alfalfa tablets. When selecting your alfalfa tablets, be sure to secure them from a good reliable source. Shaklee is my choice.

As "heart-health" maintenance, we take 1 Tablespoon daily to create the catalytic effect we desire for our hearts. In case of heart disease, arthritis, rheumatism, osteoporosis, gout or combination-conditions, such as Nan-Nan suffered, be sure to take five or six alfalfa tablets three times daily. Alfalfa helps wash out toxins that have built up over the years and adds minerals needed by the body to repair damaged cell tissue.

We often take our portion of the Dr. Rinse breakfast-mash as a tasty addition to our morning cereal. As a change of pace, we sometimes use it to top yogurt or blend it into a high-protein shake. If you don't mind a somewhat "lumpy" drink, you may also stir it into any juice, such as grape, orange, pineapple or, my favorite, cranberry.

I want to add a word here about honey. Besides being a good natural "energizer," honey is one of nature's most powerful germ killers. Harmful bacteria cannot survive in raw honey. (Editor's note: It's the bee pollen particles suspended in the raw honey that makes it a germicide. See Section III.) Primitive man made this discovery early on and used honey both as a sweet treat *and* as a salve to heal wounds. And, did you know that honey used as a sweetener doesn't result in the production of heavy body fat, as does refined sugar? Honey is delicious and digestible, as well as being nutritious. In fact, many nutrition experts consider honey a supplier of power for the heart muscle itself! If you prefer Dr. Rinse's Formula sweetened, you may add honey with a heavy hand and a clear conscience!

Once you start taking the Formula, don't be impatient! Although it is true some individuals seem to experience almost immediate relief, plan on allowing three months before the results become perceptible to you—and be pleasantly surprised if it happens sooner! After six months on the Formula, its therapeutic value will be quite apparent and you will surely be on your way to better all-around health. One final note: Authorities agree that restricting food to a low-fat diet is a good practice and will go a long way toward avoiding heart attacks, strokes and senility.

TIP: Even if you're not suffering from atherosclerosis, arthritis, hypertension (high blood pressure) or are not at-risk of cardiovascular disease, I promise the Dr. Rinse Formula will improve the quality of your health and give you so much rip-roaring energy you'll feel like a frisky kid again!

The Natural Food Alternative to

CONSTIPATION

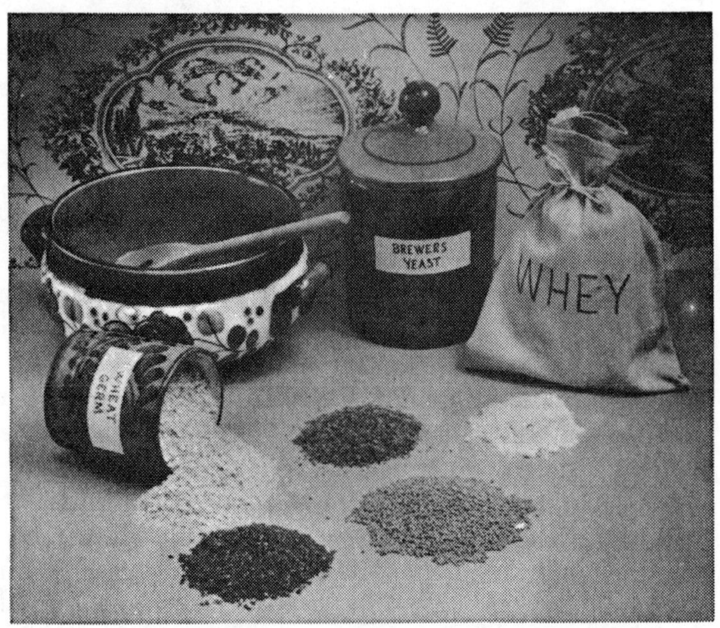

Chronic constipation is not only an often agonizing problem for many, but can also set the stage for other serious conditions of ill-health which may require medical treatment. This simple natural food and herbal kitchen recipe conquers constipation, establishes friendly intestinal flora, sweetens the bowel and encourages the peristalsis necessary for healthy normal functioning.

CONSTIPATION

The All-Too Common Problem We'd Rather Not Talk About

IN FAVOR OF FIBER—Grandmother called it "roughage" and insisted you eat your cereal and fruit every morning, your sandwich at noon and your rice and vegetables every night. Back in grandmother's day, that might have been enough. The cereals and rice were unmilled, unrefined whole-grain, so was grandmother's home-baked bread and grandmother cooked vegetables with the skins on. "Saves vitamins," she said, "and besides, you need the roughage." Grandmother was right.

Today, medical authorities call it "fiber." In fact, your doctor may have said you need more fiber (cellulose) in your diet. But adding fiber to your diet isn't as easy as it was in grandmother's day. For instance, just 4 slices of whole-grain wheat bread will provide 30 grams of fiber, probably the optimum amount we need daily, but you would have to eat *16 slices of white bread* to ingest the same 30 grams of fiber. No wonder Grampa didn't need reading material in the outhouse! His digestive system and intestinal tract most likely functioned so efficiently he didn't spend much time there!

Now, you have to shop wisely to make sure the breakfast cereal and family bread you choose is made with the whole-grain. Make sure you select natural unpolished brown rice that still retains the fiber, rather than the snowy-white variety that invariably sticks to the pan from the high starch content. Serve apples, peaches and pears unpeeled—the fiber's in the skin. Enjoy lots of high-fiber vegetables, such as beans, peas, broccoli and celery. And, for your health's's sake, cook your potatoes in the jacket and eat the skin!

FIBER—WHO NEEDS IT?—We all do. Just about everyone will most likely benefit from extra fiber in their diet. In fact, research shows most of us need from four times to *ten times* as much fiber as we normally consume daily. The average daily intake of fiber from our processed, refined, denatured foods is around 4 grams. In so-called "uncivilized" countries, the daily fiber intake averages about 30 grams, precisely the amount authorities recommend!

The intake of fiber markedly increases the growth of valuable organisms and the amount of B vitamins (particularly pantothenic acid), in the blood, urine and feces. Research shows the number of friendly intestinal bacteria are drastically decreased on a "smooth" diet lacking in fiber. Some individuals actually harbor intestinal bacteria which produce a B-complex destroying enzyme. This destructive bacteria is usually present in the stool of persons suffering from constipation.

Conditions of the digestive system and intestinal tract common to our western society include first and foremost, constipation, a national problem that continues to grow by astronomical proportions. Other disorders include appendicitis, diseases of the large intestine and rectum (including "irritable bowel syndrome"), hemorrhoids, cancer of the colon, diverticulosis and diverticulitis. Some authorities believe fiber may also affect the way in which your body processes fats and say fiber could be important in assisting to lower cholesterol levels in your blood stream. It is more than a coincidence that non-industrialized countries with a documented high-fiber intake have an enviably low incidence of these health problems.

FEAR OF FAT—As a nation, the United States is probably the most weight-conscious in the world. Literally, every third person age 16 or older is "on a diet" more or less permanently. Our books and plays, our magazines and publications, our television—and especially the advertising which continually bombards us—trumpets *"thin is in," "thin is beautiful," "thin is young,"* until we have been brainwashed into believing *only* thin is acceptable. In fact, *thin* has become a national paranoia.

In the public's collective mind, fiber equals carbohydrate, and carbohydrate equals "obesity." Nothing could be further from the truth, but it is entirely possible this erroneous thinking is the largest single contributing factor to the national problem of constipation.

FIBER IS "NO-CAL"—Your body does not digest fiber and it has no caloric or nutritional value at all. Fiber passes through the body virtually unchanged, but *supplies important bulk* needed by the intestines to carry away body wastes. This natural, bulk-producing ingredient of many foods stimulates natural intestinal movement. When your diet is deficient in fiber, your digestive process can become sluggish and you become constipated. *Fiber makes it possible for food to move through the digestive system and promotes normal intestinal function and bowel regularity.*

CONSTIPATION DEFINED—Constipation is correctly defined as the *abnormally delayed or infrequent passage of dry hardened feces.* It is important to understand that a bowel movement is *not* necessarily considered *"abnormally delayed"* if one doesn't occur naturally every day. Some persons may feel comfortable only if they evacuate their bowels daily, others may be perfectly comfortable doing so every other day and some every third day.

If the digestive system and intestinal tract are functioning correctly, the body maintains its own rhythm and doesn't require the stimulation of a laxative. It is only when the *discomfort* of an over-loaded bowel with rock-hard stool we must strain to pass occurs that we can rightly say we are constipated. Unfortunately, for too many of us, the embarrassment, discomfort and downright *pain* of constipation are a way of life.

CONSTIPATION—WHY IT OCCURS—Probably the

most common digestive disorder is gas in the intestines. Efficient digestion and freedom from gas and attendant constipation depend on the production of hydrochloric acid, bile and digestive secretions and enzymes, on the type of intestinal bacteria present and the motility (movement) of the stomach and intestines.

For instance, when we eat too much, the secretions and enzymes of the digestive tract are overwhelmed and unable to efficiently process the excess amount of food we send down to the stomach. When the amount of food eaten at one meal is efficiently digested and absorbed, none remains to support the growth of undesirable bacteria and no gas is formed.

The broad purpose of the large intestine is to conserve water. The deficiency of certain vital nutrients that decreases the motility of the intestinal muscles may allow the intestine to reabsorb too much water, resulting in a dry, hard stool. The simplest way to avoid this type of constipation is to be certain your daily intake of food and liquid includes plenty of pure unadulterated water. Some authorities recommend as much as eight 8-ounce glasses of water be taken daily.

The importance of intestinal motility cannot be overemphasized. Rhythmic contractions of the muscles in the walls of the stomach and small intestines continue for hours after we eat—mixing the food mass with digestive juices, enzymes and bile acids—and bringing already digested food into contact with the absorbing surface of the intestinal walls. Without such contractions, foods will not be efficiently digested and absorbed.

If the involuntary muscle contractions of the stomach and intestine slow down or become intermittent, undigested food stagnates for hours (or even days) and so much gas forms that suffering may become acute. When the diet has been lacking in protein, Vitamin B1, pantothenic acid and the other B vitamins for a lengthy period of time, motility is seriously restricted and constipation—or worse—results.

A potassium deficiency, for instance, causes contractions of the intestinal muscles to slow down and, if the deficiency is severe, may even cause these muscles to become partially or completely paralyzed. This condition, which creates excruciating gas pains, is also associated with agonizing constipation. Fortunately, a potassium deficiency this severe is very rare and replacing the missing nutrients increases the motility of the intestine within a day or so.

Inadequate bile flow frequently causes constipation because undigested fats react with calcium and/or iron to form hard insoluble "soaps." Permanent correction of this type of constipation lies in increasing bile production. When your diet is low in protein and simultaneously high in refined carbohydrates, little bile is produced.

If the flow of bile is insufficient—or the gall bladder doesn't empty—or the liver isn't producing sufficient bile—fats remain in such large particles that enzymes cannot combine with them. Fat digestion is then incomplete and fat absorption is seriously reduced. When hard "soaps" form, the calcium and iron in your food fail to reach the blood and this causes constipation with overly firm hard, dry stools.

Most fats from food melt at body temperature. But if bile is deficient, the melted undigested fats coat all foods and prevent the digestive enzymes from efficiently processing proteins and carbohydrates. Further, the lack of bile acids prevents the vital absorption of carotene and Vitamins A, D, E and K. People with a sluggish gall bladder are commonly found to be deficient in linoleic acid, carotene and fat-soluble vitamins.

Intestinal bacteria multiply rapidly on undigested food, releasing quantities of histamines and gas, causing gas pains, constipation, halitosis and a foul-smelling stool. If your digestion is working efficiently, a healthy individual produces stool with little or no odor.

The constipation caused by inadequate bile flow is probably the most serious of all types. If this underlying condition goes untended, it can cause severe anemia, porous bones, spontaneous fractures and the crumbling or collapse of one or more vertebrae. Faulty elimination associated with gall bladder problems invariably indicates a major loss of vital minerals.

Spastic constipation, characterized by spasms in the large bowel, is documented to occur when deficiencies of calcium, magnesium, potassium and Vitamin B6 are combined with other nutrient deficiencies which result in faulty elimination. A lack of choline, essential to liver function and one of the B complex vitamins, has been shown to produce constipation. Other symptoms of choline deficiency, such as unexplained headaches, dizziness, ear noises and heart palpitations usually improve or disappear completely within ten days of adequate choline supplementation.

In the case of atonic (lack of physiological tone, especially of a contractile organ), colon, poor muscle tone interferes with the circulation of blood, slows normal lymph flow, inhibits digestion—and often causes constipation. Weak and inefficiently functioning muscles may even make it impossible to control urination or a bowel movement, resulting in an embarrassing accident. Weak muscles cannot properly support internal organs—and organs not adequately supported cannot perform their functions efficiently.

As muscles consist largely of layers of protein (with some essential fatty acids), these nutrients must be present in sufficient amounts to maintain muscle strength. However, the chemistry of the muscles themselves and the nerves which control them is so complex just about every nutrient known plays a part in their contraction, relaxation and repair.

When lack of muscle tone results in fatigue, gas distention and constipation (and perphaps even the inability to pass urine without a catheter), the taking of potassium chloride tablets (and Vitamin E supplementation) have proved effective. However, the average adult obtains ample potassium in his diet from fruits and vegetables, particularly cooked green leafy ones, and by avoiding refined foods.

An often-overlooked cause of chronic constipation is a psychoneurosis wherein the mind produces such anxiety the individual is unable to move the bowels. Well-nourished adults on excellent diets may sometimes suffer from digestive disturbances resulting in a serious and long-standing problem with constipation. When these individuals are closely questioned under the care of a psychiatrist, they are often discovered to feel lonely and unloved and, in most instances, had severe colic as a baby. The unconscious mind recreates the "colic" that brought love and attention to the child. Treatment may be with sedatives, tranquilizers or psychotherapy.

An obstruction is anything which interferes with the passage of the intestinal contents through the bowel. Fortunately, the most common cause is adhesions left over from a prior surgery. Symptoms are cramping and severe, sharp abdominal pain with distention and vomiting. If the obstruction has not completely closed the bowel off, this condition may respond to aspiration of the bowel contents with a long intestinal tube. If aspiration does not clear the obstruction promptly, surgery is necessary.

On the very extreme side, constipation may be a sign of obstruction of the colon caused by a tumor or cancer. Fortunately, malignant tumors are more rare than benign tumors, but both produce the same symptoms and both are treated by surgery. However, if constipation continues to the point where the individual is unable to pass anything and is in real pain, a complete physical examination and x-ray of the colon is very much in order.

A little-recognized side-effect of long-term constipation may be the development of varicose veins and hemorrhoids. In fact, some researchers believe the major cause of varicose veins is actually faulty elimination. When an overloaded bowel presses against veins in the lower abdomen year after year, the valves in the veins gradually break down allowing a reverse flow of blood.

In peoples of the world eating a diet of unrefined, mostly raw foods, varicose veins and hemorrhoids (actually a form of varicose veins), are virtually unknown. Among the Zulus in Africa, for instance, only three persons in a population of 115,319 were found to have varicose veins while 10% of the entire population of Britain suffers from this unsightly and uncomfortable condition.

Scientists believe a return to the old ways of eating can help prevent, or even correct, the situation. A hundred years ago, the diet might conceivably have consisted of fruits, vegetables (mostly raw), meats, eggs, cheese, sour milks (acidopholous/yogurt), nuts and whole-grain breads and cereals with no refined or processed foods at all. This wholesome diet would surely prevent constipation as well.

Some lower abdominal pain may easily be confused with constipation. As a case in point, irritable colon, spastic colon and spastic colitis are medical terms and all refer to the same condition, which is functional and not organic. A common cause of lower abdominal pain is the irritable colon syndrome. Symptoms may include a cramping in the abdomen, bloating, the passing of gas and an uncomfortable distension of the area.

Once the diagnosis is confirmed, treatment of an irritable colon consists of reassuring the patient the condition is not serious, advising a bland diet and, occasionally, prescribing sedatives or tranquilizers. When intestinal gas or bloating is severe, relief is often obtained by use of a gas-relieving silicone derivative. Mucous colitis is merely a variation of the irritable colon syndrome with the same symptoms as outlined above, except a large amount of harmless mucus is passed with the bowel movement.

In its early stages, appendicitis mimics constipation. As the condition escalates, symptoms include nausea, vomiting and severe abdominal pain. The abdominal muscles become rigid and are very tender to the touch, with any pressure causing much pain. Body temperature rises and the number of white cells in the body increases. An accurate diagnosis must be made by a physician on the basis of x-ray and white blood cell count.

RELATED CONDITIONS—Diverticulosis is a condition in which small pockets form on the colonic wall. Numerous small pockets may occur which give the appearance of grapes. These sacs form in a weakened area of the bowel wall, weakened somewhat as a balloon or inner-tube may have a thin area. Diverticulosis can be diagnosed only by an x-ray examination and is most common in persons who are constantly constipated and must strain to pass their stool. Unless a complication occurs, no treatment is necessary.

Diverticulitis is an inflammation or infection in one or more of the diverticulosis sacs. Symptoms are low, cramping abdominal pain, which may be mistaken in its early stages for constipation. If the condition progresses, chills and fever and even the development of a mass which produces an obstruction in the bowel can occur.

Again, diagnosis can only be made by x-ray. Treatment of acute diverticulitis consists of antibiotics and a liquid diet. Individuals who suffer from chronic diverticulitis must eat properly and work to develop good bowel habits. If symptoms persist or an obstruction occurs, surgery is indicated.

In the foregoing pages, we have only briefly examined the many causes of constipation. To go into a complete and medically technical run-down of the workings of the stomach, intestines and bowel, would take a book in itself. Suffice it to say that the digestive system, intestinal tract, colon and rectum collectively—and, for the most part, very efficiently—processes the food we eat, extracts the nutrients we need to function and then excretes the waste matter.

I am just now reminded of a delightful old gentleman I knew years ago. He had a pink and shiny bald head with a monk's fringe of white hair and an enormous old-fashioned handlebar moustache slightly yellowing at the ends. He was known in the neighborhood as "The Colonel," but his true name escapes me now.

I enjoyed chatting with him. The Colonel hadn't lost his sense of humor and his mind was as sharp as a tack. However, at 72 years of age, he suffered most dreadfully with chronic constipation and constantly groused his "digestive juices were all used up along with all the other juices that made life worth living." In the twilight of his life, he existed almost entirely on liquids and told me once, "At my age, a good bowel movement is better and more satisfying than sex ever was, at least as I remember it!"

If you are a sufferer of chronic constipation, you might echo that sentiment at times. Don't despair, dear reader, help is on the way! In the following sections we will explore the various types of laxative remedies and I will give you a kitchen recipe guaranteed to keep the pipes open and in good working order. Read on.

LET'S TALK LAXATIVES

There Must be a Better Way

If you suffer from occasional constipation, you may be one of the many who ignore the condition in the hope it will go away. True, nature has a way of taking care of the problem and, if we just let nature take it's course, relief may be just a day or so away. Or it may not.

On the other hand, the constipation may be so acute—and so painful—that the only answer seems to be to resort to a laxative that will relieve the problem. Judging by the sale of over-the-counter laxatives, this is the solution the majority of us favor.

More than 5,000 types of laxatives and cathartics are used in the United States alone. Americans spend more than a hundred million dollars per year on various treatments for constipation. Many of these laxatives contain harsh and even poisonous substances to cause the colon to react and eliminate them as rapidly as possible—and the fecal material along with them.

When the body is functioning properly, the food we consume passes through the stomach and small intestine in a relatively short period of time. The length of time required for passage through the large intestine is all-important. We want to hurry it along. When the movement of waste material slows down and becomes sluggish, harmful bacteria builds up and the mass can putrify. In many persons, the passage is too slow and constipation results.

Good bowel habits are essential to promote a clean digestive tract. Normal intestinal function demands we allow the bowels to move when they will. It may surprise you to know that the lower end of the intestine is of a size that requires emptying every six hours. However, through habit, most of us have trained our bodies to retain waste for 24-hours or more. When nature calls, the urge should be answered quickly to avoid developing the bad bowel habits which lead to constipation.

Constipation is so common that about half the adults in the United States suffer from this condition, either as a chronic complaint or as a once-in-awhile problem. Because it is so common, most of us feel we know enough about it and usually treat ourselves with an overnight laxative—but the use of laxatives in itself can also create problems.

LAXATIVE DEFINED—The term *laxative* comes from the Latin and literally means "having a tendency *to loosen* or relax, specifically to relieve constipation." But far too many laxatives, instead of *loosening* or *relaxing*, work on the "blast out" theory. They create an overpowering urge and the bowel expels its contents, usually hard and sizable, without regard for the relative lack of elasticity of the rectum. (Ouch!) Let's examine the various types of laxatives available.

MINERAL OIL—For more than 25 years, the American Medical Association has been preaching against the use of mineral oil, probably the most damaging of all laxatives in use. Yet some unenlightened physicians still prescribe it and many take it routinely for constipation because of its lubricating action. Consider these facts: Mineral oil decreases the body's ability to absorb calcium and phosphorus and mineral oil itself absorbs vitamins A, D. E, K and carotene from the nutrients in the intestines. In addition, mineral oil picks up the fat-soluble vitamins from liquids and tissues throughout the body. All these valuable vitamins are then excreted and lost.

STIMULANT LAXATIVES—Castor oil and laxatives containing *phenolphthalein* are considered stimulant (or contact) laxatives and work directly on the small intestine to promote a bowel movement. These purge-type laxatives are often used for complete bowel evacuation prior to x-ray or surgery and usually prior to an endoscopic examination of the colon as well. Occasional use under a doctor's care is necessary and not harmful, but regular home-use can cause an excessive loss of water and body salts, resulting in a weakening of the body. Many popular over-the-counter laxatives are too harsh to be used regularly as self-treatment.

SALINE LAXATIVES—The old familiar standbys *milk of magnesia* and *epsom salts* are typical examples of saline type laxatives. This type laxative is attractive as it often produces rapid results just when we need it most. However, their action is too thorough and over-empties the bowel. What happens then? Because the bowel is empty, several days pass before a normal bowel movement is necessary. This sets the stage for a self-induced condition known as *rebound constipation.*

REBOUND CONSTIPATION—When occasional constipation occurs and one of the popular over-the-counter laxatives is taken, which usually completely evacuates the bowel, having a normal bowel movement the following day is an impossibility. The body may require as much as several days to extract nutrients and process waste matter before we once again feel an urge to move our bowels. It's important to understand this time-lag which commonly occurs after taking a laxative is *not* constipation, but just nature catching up after the body's normal routine is interrupted. Don't let *rebound constipation* fool you into taking another laxative the following day.

LAXATIVE ABUSE—Individuals who have the idea that it's not only necessary but *normal* to have a daily bowel movement are likely candidates for laxative abuse. This thinking can lead to over-frequent self-dosing with laxatives, which results in a lazy bowel. In time, bowel habits become abnormal and may even cease to function *without* the stimulation of a laxative.

THE DANGERS OF LAXATIVES—Abnormal bowel habits, described above, are not the only problems arising from the constant use of laxatives. Repeated misuse can lead to dehydration (excessive loss of water), loss of nutrients (proteins and vitamins), and loss of electrolytes (body salts), such as sodium, potassium and calcium. Further, laxative abuse has been shown to cause spastic colitis, gastrointestinal disturbances and even physical changes in the intestine leading to chronic diarrhea.

WHEN *NOT* TO TAKE A LAXATIVE—The occasional use of a laxative is not normally harmful, but there are certain times when laxatives *must not* be taken. If stomach cramps, nausea, vomiting or other symptoms of appendicitis are present, *do not* take any type laxative. If you do have appendicitis, stimulating bowel activity with a laxative could result in the rupture of an inflamed appendix.

INTESTINAL MANAGEMENT—Many authorities believe the most important thing we can do for our bodies is to adopt a health-building routine that promotes a clean intestinal tract. Some of the most important life-functions take place in the intestines. Waste material not regularly evacuated can accumulate and the toxic by-products of putrefaction can be carried by the blood and lymph to every part of the body. There is a strong relationship between the cleanliness and health of the intestinal tract and the health of the body as a whole.

Establishing normal intestinal flora with normal bacterial activity is of primary importance to establishing normal bowel movements. The simple kitchen recipe for a natural food-laxative in the following pages is *the better way* for cleansing and revitalizing the bowel and conquering constipation forever!

THE BETTER WAY

The Natural-Food Antidote for Constipation

Babies do it. Birds do it. Animals do it and the natural-living so-called "uncivilized" peoples of the world do it. Anyone who has ever cared for a baby has to be aware of the sounds of satisfaction the little one gives forth as he fills his diaper after eating. The native disappears into the bush or jungle and returns relieved. The dog barks and scratches the door to go out after his dinner. Nature intended that we evacuate our bowels a short time after each meal. But—*most of us don't do it.*

Instead, for whatever the reason, far too many of us put nature "on-hold" until a more convenient time. We may be away from home and dislike using a public facility. We may be in an important business meeting. We may be involved in a lengthy telephone call. We may be on the tennis court or playing softball at the company picnic. We may be stirring jelly or a pudding on the stove that might burn. We may even be intensely interested in a television program and wait for a commercial before making a mad dash for the commode where we try to fit nature's call into a 2-minute station break.

Some authorities believe that over 90% of the "diseases of civilization" are fostered by improper functioning of the colon. In fact, many well-accredited sources believe a sluggish colon gives rise to conditions as widely diverse as appendicitis, tonsilitis, infections of the liver and gall-bladder, dysfunction of the heart and blood vessels, sinusitis, arthritis and even rheumatism. This century has seen an astounding increase in the number of surgeries and treatments for the various parts of and problems of the colon, including the rectum and the anus itself. Consider hemorrhoids, fistulas, the prostate and the killer—cancer.

Our modern way of life is a major contributing factor. Instead of a plain, natural diet, we now eat highly refined and demineralized foods, often on the run. We are subjected daily to the stress and strain of surviving on the "fast-track" in our highly "civilized" world. We're too "busy" getting on to take adequate exercise. And, possible most important, we are otherwise occupied or we are too "polite" (or too self-conscious) to excuse ourselves when nature signals a need to evacuate our bowels and promptly take care of the situation.

When toxic waste matter is left to stagnate in the lower bowel tract, the system becomes polluted and constipation (or worse) results. In time, a condition of peristaltic malfunction occurs in the bowel with the fecal matter becoming condensed and compressed and movements are infrequent and difficult. Peristalsis is "nature calling," the rhythmic waves of involuntary contraction of the intestines which forces waste matter through the passageway and out. Inconvenient or not, more and more medical researchers are saying we would be better off to emulate the natives and move our bowels as often as we eat a regular meal.

(Incidentally, speaking of the natives and their healthy bowel habits for a moment, you might find it as fascinating as I do to know that certain tribes in Africa who eat with their fingers from a common pot have a stiff penalty for the individual who "forgets" and dips into the pot with his left hand—the hand is immediately chopped off! (This may be primitive, but it's a highly effective method of sanitation.) Why? *Only the right hand is for eating.* The left hand is for wiping the behind with a handful of leaves after the trip into the bush.)

Certainly all of the foregoing material has impressed on you the importance of a healthy intestinal tract. Fortunately, it's not impossible to correct a lifetime history of chronic constipation, a sluggish colon and abnormal bowel habits. In fact, the remedy we're going to lay out for you now will vanquish constipation forever and may even give you a new lease on life! I call it:

THE ANTIDOTE TO CONSTIPATION

This old recipe, which I have updated for ease of preparation with today's ingredients, was developed by my doctor-father, who preferred to treat his patients with natural herbs whenever possible. He used this traditional country remedy for many, many years in his practice with great success. Unlike chemical laxatives, this combination of natural ingredients can be used every day without the least harm or side-effects to the body. My family still takes it regularly and many of our friends have used it for years. It always works wonders!

I have named it the "antidote," because an antidote is something that relieves, prevents or counteracts the effects of poison. "Poison" is defined as something that through its chemical action kills, injures or impairs an organism, something destructive or harmful, an object of aversion or abhorrence, something that inhibits the activity of or course of a reaction or process. This *antidote* will relieve, prevent and counteract the effects of the *constipation* which may be *poisoning* our system. In short, this is the perfect description of this recipe and I'm delighted with it.

We want to avoid the need for the quick temporary relief provided by laxatives, enemas and colonics. We want to cleanse, feed and stimulate the intestinal tract to allow it to work normally and naturally on its own without outside interference. Using the proper natural foods, we will build up the body, clean it out and encourage the necessary peristaltic action to allow the bowels to work freely and properly. And that's just what The

Antidote can do for you.

The first order of business in cleansing and revitalizing the bowel is to establish friendly intestinal flora. In any type of intestinal disorder, the intestinal bacteria needs normalizing. Without normal bacterial activity, we may suffer a gas attack, diarrhea, constipation or set ourselves up for the onset of serious disease. The healthy way to supply the body with friendly bacteria is by adding a *lactic-acid* product, such as whey or yogurt, to your daily diet.

WHEY—Whey, the watery part of milk left when the curds are removed, is rich in lactose, minerals and vitamins and contains lactalbumin and traces of fat. Whey is needed to feed the friendly bacteria in the intestines and colon, keeping it healthy and active, and to "sweeten" the bowel. It may be produced from either goats' or cows' milk and can be fresh or powdered. For our purposes, the Antidote contains powdered whey.

Fermented milks have been used as foods and beverages in many cultures for centuries. It is the action of *bacillus acidi lactiti* which causes milk to sour. When the bacilli convert the milk sugar into lactic acid, the growth of disease-producing bacteria ceases and the milk becomes more digestible in the bargain. Lactic acid is a strong neutralizer of putrefaction in the colon.

To demonstrate the neutralizing power of lactic acid, a researcher immersed a pound of tainted beef in a crock of buttermilk. After just a few days in the buttermilk, bacteriological examination showed no putrefactive bacteria present in the meat. Science has shown that disease-producing bacteria cannot thrive in an acid medium, proving the desirability of adding lactic-acid to the diet. *You will find whey powder is a prime ingredient of The Antidote.*

YEAST—Yeast contains almost no fat, starch or sugar and its excellent protein sticks to your ribs, satisfies the appetite and increases your basal metabolism. In fact, more nutrients are concentrated in yeast than in almost any other food. (Only bee pollen beats yeast in complete nutrient content. See Section III.) Good nutrition is a necessity in overcoming constipation forever. Research has shown that a deficiency of certain nutrients can in itself be a cause of constipation.

The B vitamin *inositol* is a case in point. A hundred times *more* inositol than any other vitamin (except niacin) is found in the human body. Inositol is so important in the diet that when animals are put on a regimen lacking inositol, their hair falls out, they develop an eczema rash (dermatitis), abnormalities of the eyes (inositol is concentrated in the lens of the human eye)—and severe *constipation*. The good news is that all these conditions clear up when the diet is supplemented with inositol. Yeast is a particularly good source of inositol.

Yeast also is rich in *choline*, another B vitamin, which has many duties in the body. It is necessary for the synthesis of nucleic acid and for the production of DNA and RNA. A deficiency of choline has been shown to result in high blood pressure and accompanying strokes, hemorrhages of the eyes and nephritis (kidney disease). When individuals suffering from a lack of choline have been adequately supplied, headaches, dizziness, ear noises and *constipation* improved or disappeared within 5 to 10 days, with the blood pressure dropping to normal.

Although *niacin* is somewhat difficult to obtain in a normal diet, yeast is an excellent source. A person laboring under a niacin deficiency usually experiences persistent *constipation*. Simultaneously, anemia and digestive disturbances are apparent, as the stomach cannot produce sufficient enzymes, digestive juices and stomach acid for normal digestion. The intestinal tract is stressed and constipation can alternate with diarrhea. If the niacin deficiency continues, the individual exhibits personality changes and may become depressed and hostile.

A lack of *thiamin,* vitamin B1, causes digestive disturbances in a number of ways. Energy production is so faulty that contractions of the stomach and peristalsis slows down. The stomach can't produce the necessary hydrochloric acid for the normal digestive processes, proteins are incompletely digested, minerals stay insoluble and several vitamins are completely destroyed. Gas pain, flatulence and *constipation* are inevitable. If thiamin is not supplied quickly, more serious conditions result. Yeast supplies the thiamin the body requires.

Persons on a refined, denatured diet deficient in *potassium* quickly develop fatigue, listlessness, gas pains, *constipation,* insomnia and low blood sugar. Muscles become soft and flabby and the pulse becomes slow, weak and irregular. By far the greatest harm caused by a lack of potassium is the effect on the heart. Heart attacks are often associated with a low potassium intake. An excessive intake of sodium (salt) can produce a potassium deficiency even when it appears the diet is adequately supplied. Yeast is an incomparable source of needed potassium.

To sum it all up, yeast is a rich and concentrated source of complete protein, the B vitamins (inositol, choline and thiamin), niacin and the minerals (particularly potassium) necessary for normal peristalsis and clean intestinal functioning. *As you can see, yeast plays a very important part in the Antidote formula.*

WHEAT GERM—Although there are many varieties of wheat, the first true wheat plant came from the lands of Galilee in Israel. All the hundreds of varieties of wheat grown around the world are descended from this original grain, mentioned favorably many times in religious writings. The germ of wheat is a strengthening food for all animals, including man, and is a source of natural vitamins and minerals. The germ is particularly rich in Vitamins E and B and, like yeast, contains inositol, choline, niacin and thiamin. *Besides being good for you all over, wheat germ is specified in the Antidote formula to nurture the friendly acidophilous culture.*

PSYLLIUM SEEDS—In herbal lore, *psyllium* is considered a superior intestinal lubricant and aid to the digestive tract. As a hydrophilic mucilloid, psyllium is often recommended by physicians because it is gentle,effective and virtually without the harmful side effects of chemical laxatives. Psyllium provides bulk (Grandmother's "roughage") with natural dietary fiber and absorbs large quantities of water to form a gel which softens the stool. Psyllium creates a soft, formed easy-to-pass stool with no cramping or accidents. Psyllium is considered to be an excellent colon and intestinal cleanser and healer, strengthening and toning the tissues. It does not irritate the mucous membranes and the intestinal tract is nicely lubricated for a smooth passage. *With these outstanding qualities, you might expect to find psyllium in the Antidote.* It is.

FLAXSEED—Flaxseed is another favorite of the master herbalists of the last century. It is a soothing natural laxative and provides additional fiber. Flaxseed can stimulate peristalsis and the glandular secretions necessary to normal intestinal functioning. This herb is so gentle, it has been given to sickly babies for its blood enriching properties. It is said to heal the body as it nourishes and is soothing to the throat, the linings of the intestines and the entire digestive tract. *Flaxseed is included in the Antidote for its healing qualities and gentle laxative action.*

In addition, these two important herbs are said to aid in cleansing waste matter from the liver, gall ducts and alimentary canal. Both psyllium and flaxseed encourage necessary bile secretions into the duodenum and help normalize the peristaltic action of the bowels.

MUSTARD SEED—Animals in the wild instinctively seek out and eat the mustard plant, presumably recognizing it for the fine tonic, disinfectant and digestive aid it is. Mustard seeds promote a healthy appetite, stimulate salivation (saliva acts upon food as we chew and is the first part of the digestive process) and the secretion of vital digestive juices. *Mustard seed helps eliminate intestinal gas and, with its other properties, this powerful little herb is an excellent optional addition to the Antidote.*

Experiments with animals have proved an unbalanced diet shortens the lifespan in one way or another. Indications continue to accumulate showing that an improper diet may actually shorten the life expectancy of man as well. Establishing a pattern of constipation and the resultant over-use of laxatives which leads to abnormal functioning of the intestinal tract is just one way we abuse our bodies. The food we eat, its type, its elements and the amounts in which we take it, have a profound effect on our body, our intestinal tract, our degree of health and well-being and our general fitness.

The natural way of conquering constipation forever is the major objective of The Natural-Food Antidote for Constipation—and that's just what it will do for you. I have attempted to analyze this recipe as completely as possible and my analysis shows that the specific nutrients required to cleanse and sweeten the bowel, encourage peristalsis and establish (or re-establish) good bowel habits are present in the formula.

Bon appetit!

THE NATURAL FOOD ANTIDOTE FOR CONSTIPATION

1 cup Whey Powder
1 1/2 cups Brewer's Yeast
1 cup Wheat Germ
1/2 cup Psyllium Seeds
1/2 cup Flaxseed
1/2 cup Mustard Seed*

(*Mustard Seed may be eliminated if not readily available)

All of these ingredients can be easily purchased at your local health-food store—or try a country co-op for lower prices. Both wheat germ and Brewer's yeast can be used in flake or powder form, but do purchase the whole seeds. Psyllium seeds, flaxseed and mustard seed should not be *powdered*, but *used whole.*

Simply mix thoroughly with your spoon in a big bowl until the blend is uniform. We suggest you mix up a two to four week supply (1 to 2 pounds). The mixture stores well in a plastic bag (with a twist tie) or jar, but always keep the lid tight. (The above recipe will produce an approximate 2 week supply for two people.)

Place 1 or 2 tablespoons of the mixture in a cup with the beverage of your choice (tea, milk, coffee or water) and swallow slowly. Additional liquid is advisable. Always rinse down with a second glass of your favorite drink. Or just put a spoonful in your mouth and wash it down with plenty of liquid.

We suggest you take one or two tablespoons before meals, depending on your condition. You be the judge. Allow one or two days for results. Remember, this is *not* an overnight chemical blast, but a gentle *food* laxative that will correct faulty bowel habits and conquer constipation forever. In the beginning, it may take two or three days before a normal healthy bowel movement is evident.

This Natural Food Laxative is also a very fine health breakfast. It is low in calories, easy on your stomach and helps prevent indigestion, as well as encouraging peristalsis of the intestines and promoting bowel regularity. This mixture of special stool-softening herbal ingredients activates the intestines and supports the natural, normal functioning of the bowel.

Tip: Authorities agree eating foods raw or lightly cooked, using whole grain breads and cereals rather than bleached white flour products, taking complex carbohydrates with natural sugars (fruits rather than pastries) and drinking plenty of water daily to flush out impurities will go a long way toward fixing whatever ails us—including constipation!